"In *But I Deserve This Chocolate!*, Susan Albers insightfully points out our fifty best diet-derailing excuses and shows one or two easy ways to tackle each excuse. The result is a punchy, inspiring book that is full of new ideas and practical tips for getting us past our most diet-destroying excuses. Fifty cheers!"

> —Brian Wansink, PhD, professor and director of Cornell University Food and Brand Lab and author of *Mindless Eating*

"These tips can spur you toward success on your personal health journey by teaching you how to make your thoughts work for you."

> —Ashley Koff, RD, dietitian and author of *Mom Energy*

"Changing how we think about food, eating, our weight, and our bodies is a critical step in successfully overcoming struggles with eating and weight. *But I Deserve This Chocolate!* offers a wealth of practical exercises that can help end common thoughts that keep us stuck in such struggles. It's a logical and easy-to-use addition to Susan Albers' valuable series on mindful eating. We're grateful to have this new resource for the women who come to us for help."

> —Marsha Hudnall, MS, RD, director and owner of Green Mountain at Fox Run, a women's retreat for healthy living without dieting

"*But I Deserve This Chocolate!* sheds the clear light of reason on mindful eating."

> —Patrick Fanning, coauthor of *Mind and Emotions* and *Self-Esteem*

"With Albers' newest book, we learn how mindful eating is like jumping into a chilly pool on a hot summer day: Dipping your toe in might feel uncomfortable, but once you dive in, you never want to leave. She compassionately guides, challenges, educates, and empowers readers. You think you deserve chocolate? You deserve this book."

> —Leslie Goldman, author of *Locker Room Diaries: The Naked Truth About Women, Body Image, and Re-imagining the 'Perfect' Body*

"Giving the body what it needs is the foundation of self-care, whether your body needs nutrition, movement, sleep, relaxation, or even chocolate. When we meet these needs in a mindful way, we take away the power of the internal critic that can often derail our ability to find overall wellness. Susan Albers' easy-to-understand mindfulness methods will fully engage readers who are interested in balanced, healthy eating."

> —Chevese Turner, CEO and founder, Binge Eating Disorder Association (BEDA)

"But I deserve this chocolate!"

THE 50 MOST COMMON DIET-DERAILING EXCUSES AND HOW TO OUTWIT THEM

SUSAN ALBERS, PsyD

New Harbinger Publications, Inc.

Distributed in Canada by Raincoast Books

Copyright © 2011 by Susan Albers
New Harbinger Publications, Inc.
5674 Shattuck Avenue
Oakland, CA 94609
www.newharbinger.com

Cover design by Amy Shoup
Text design by Michele Waters-Kermes
Acquired by Catharine Meyers
Edited by Nelda Street

Library of Congress Cataloging in Publication Data on file

13		12		11							
10	9	8	7	6	5	4	3	2	1		

First printing

This book is printed with soy ink.

FSC
www.fsc.org
MIX
Paper from
responsible sources
FSC® C011825

To Brooklyn and Jack.
See you at the Plaza.

Contents

Contents

Acknowledgments

We are what we think.
All that we are arises with our thoughts.
With our thoughts, we make our world.
　　—Buddha

To those who are always in my thoughts: Brooklyn Bowling, Jack Bowling, John Bowling, Jane Lindquist Lesniewski, Betsy Beyer Swope, Dr. Jason Grief, Eric Lingenfelter and Dr. Bronwyn Wilke Lingenfelter, Linda Serotta, Dr. Angie Albers, Dr. Eric Brooks, Dr. Thomas Albers, John Bowling, and

Jimmer Bowling. A special thanks to J. R. for holding down the fort so I could type to my heart's content. Thanks to Susan Heady for her feedback on this manuscript. Many thanks to Rhonda Bowling for being "Nani" and Carmela Albers for being "Mimi." As always, I am so grateful for and can't believe my good fortune in finding such a good friend in Dr. Victoria Gould.

Thanks to New Harbinger editors Catharine Meyers and Jess Beebe. Your ideas and feedback are always greatly appreciated. Thanks to Earlita Chenault for her efforts in promoting my books so that they could reach all those who are interested in mindful eating. Finally, I'd like to thank the readers and my clients who continue to show me every day how important and life changing mindful eating can be.

Welcome

A crust eaten in peace is better than a banquet partaken in anxiety.

—Aesop

Consider how you would finish this statement: "I can't start eating healthy today because..." Every one of us could complete this sentence with ten different explanations: "I don't have time." "I'm too stressed out." "I have too much going on right now." "I have PMS; I need chocolate!" Your mind can come up with some pretty creative ways to justify comfort eating and to avoid eating in a mindful, balanced, healthy way.

If you picked up this book, you probably want to lose weight or improve your eating habits. In fact, you may desire nothing more than to eat healthier. Then why is it so easy to find a million reasons to avoid doing so? Why do you fall for excuses every time? Rest assured, it is *not* because you're lazy or unable to change.

The Paradox: Why Don't I Make the Changes I Want to Make?

Here's a way to consider the paradox of wanting to improve your eating but thinking up every excuse not to do so. Imagine that it's the perfect day for swimming. As you approach the pool, you see kids and adults soaring off the diving board, and then laughing and splashing around happily. You ask, "Is the water warm?" A person responds from the water, "Come on in. It's really cold at first, but then it's great." This is disappointing. You hoped the water would be warm, like bathwater, so you could easily jump in.

For a moment, you place your toe in the water but quickly pull it out. It's extremely cold! You notice your mind kicking into gear: *I can't do this. It's too cold.* You try to find reasons not to go in right now: *Well, maybe I'll wait until it warms up* or *I'm not quite ready to jump in yet.*

Changing your eating habits is like entering the pool. Though it's something you want to do and would really enjoy once you got into it, you're reluctant at first. You find excuses to avoid the very first sensations you would feel. But, as with the pool, you would quickly acclimate if you got all the way in. Too often, people put only a toe into mindful eating to try it out, but then quickly pull it right back out. Making direct contact with the cold water and staying with it allows you to acclimate to it. Then, you stop thinking about the temperature and just enjoy it. With time you won't think of mindful eating as a new or different behavior. In fact, you'll take pleasure in it.

If you tend to get paralyzed or can't push past the excuses in your head, this is the book for you. You'll learn skillful ways to respond to these self-sabotaging thoughts. But it's only fair to warn you: This book contains some radical and surprising information. What you are about to read will go against the grain of much of what you know about traditional dieting. Most fad diets tell you to "control" your eating, use willpower, ignore your cravings, or just stop eating. Recall for a moment where this got you in the past. Feeling frustrated or hopeless? Maybe it led you to make more excuses? Perhaps you're thinking *I need to get control.* This is a sign that the diet mentality may be deeply ingrained in you. Rest assured that there are alternatives to fad dieting and trying to "control" your body.

The approach you'll learn in this book is entirely unique, which is good news. If you want different results, you have to do something new. Too often, we try the same approach over and over again, expecting something different to happen, particularly with diets. Thankfully, there are other ways to stop wrestling with your hunger and wagging your finger at yourself for being "bad" whenever you eat treats and other tasty food.

Introduction

Have you ever wondered why you have every intention of eating in a healthy, mindful way but then don't do it? You get up in the morning and make firm plans to eat healthier but, by noon, tell yourself *I don't have time* or *I'll start tomorrow*. Despite your best efforts to eat healthy types and portions of food, you get stuck and fall back into old habits. One important factor that may be standing in the way of change is the way you think.

This book is about overcoming mindless thinking, or thinking in habitual and automatic ways, which sabotages healthy eating. Routine and automatic ways of thinking lead to what I call "gridlock thinking." Like the road in a traffic jam, your mind can get congested when thoughts come at you from all directions. Some thoughts urge you to eat healthfully, while others tell you to indulge. The competing demands lock you in place so that you can't move forward, which can be incredibly frustrating and irritating—just like being stuck in traffic.

Getting past your thoughts is trickier than you might guess. Thinking can take place below your awareness, like background music. Although you may not consciously "hear" your thoughts, they play a significant part in determining what you do and don't eat. Thoughts that push you away rather than toward your goals pop up effortlessly, beyond your control. When you think the same way for many years, the habitual nature of your thought patterns is hard to break. Imagine if one day you decided to drive an entirely different route to work or school, even though you've driven the same route for many years. It could take a few days or months before driving in the new direction became second nature.

Though there are many types of thoughts, there are two slippery slopes toward gridlock thinking: excuses and self-judgments. Excuses sound like *I don't have time to eat healthy* or *I don't have the energy*. It's easy to think of a hundred different reasons why you can't start right now. Often excuses and procrastination aren't about being "lazy," but serve a hidden function that you will learn more about in this book.

Self-judgment is the second type of thought that leads to ` thinking. It is the critical commentary in your head `ly evaluates what and how you eat: *You're bad if you* ` r You've ruined it anyway, so why not?* Unfortunately,

2

this tactic doesn't inspire you to change. In fact, it pushes you further into gridlock, setting up a mental roadblock.

You will acquire two new skills in this book: First, you'll learn mindfulness skills, which will help you spot excuses and learn how to stop falling for them. Second, you'll discover a new way to talk to yourself that focuses on compassion and motivation rather than scolding yourself for your eating errors. These two skills will help you get back on the road to mindful eating.

Why I Wrote This Book

To confess, I love writing about mindful eating. I write or blog about this subject almost daily. Why? Because I truly believe that mindful eating is healing, and importantly, there's research to support it.

There's another reason why I wrote this book. I noticed something very interesting each time I gave a mindful-eating workshop, talked to readers, and worked directly with clients. The majority of people struggling with healthy, mindful eating convey remarkably similar thoughts. Sometimes people even relate the same statements verbatim, such as, "I blew my diet, and now I can't get back on track," or "I feel so guilty when I eat." After many years of hearing the same thoughts that sabotage mindful eating, I began to keep track of the most common ones. Although there are many more, this book compiles frequently stated self-sabotaging thoughts. I want to share with you creative and mindful ways to talk "with," rather than "to," yourself to prevent gridlock thinking.

Who Is This Book For?

Whether you're a man or woman, teen or adult, this book is for you if you are trying to eat more mindfully, manage your weight, lose weight, or take charge of your eating habits. You'll be particularly interested in this book if:

- You think *Today is the day I'll start eating healthy* but then find excuses or have difficulty getting started.

- You keep promising yourself *Tomorrow I'll start eating healthier* or *I'll go jogging tomorrow* but almost never do. Procrastinating about making changes is a problem for you.

- You get started eating healthy but easily get off track. Once you're off track, you feel as if you've blown it, and can't see how to get back on the path to healthy eating.

- You tend to overthink things, easily being swayed by your thoughts, particularly those that talk you out of eating mindfully.

- You find it difficult to get motivated. A bad day or a negative thought can kill your momentum.

- You have a very critical inner voice that judges what you do and don't eat.

- You think about food a significant portion of your day, to the extent of interfering with other important tasks.

- You have a lot of important reasons to improve your health, like a diagnosis of diabetes or high cholesterol. Despite knowing this, you still can't seem to get started.

The Eating Mindfully Book Series

But I Deserve This Chocolate! The Fifty Most Common Diet-Derailing Excuses and How to Outwit Them is the fifth book I've written on mindful eating. If you're wondering whether this book has something new to offer, the answer is yes! Although I introduced how to be mindful of your thoughts in my first book, *Eating Mindfully: How to End Mindless Eating and Enjoy a Balanced Relationship with Food*, this book delves deeper into how your mind works. Thoughts have a lot of power and can make or break your eating habits.

This book is great, whether you're a beginner or a more-advanced mindful eater. If you're just getting started, this is a helpful place to begin. Thoughts affect behavior, so it may be useful to understand how you think before trying to change your behavior. Use this book as a launchpad to get you started. Even if we are well versed in mindful, healthy eating, none of us is immune to the sneaky little thoughts urging us to eat mindlessly on holidays or whenever we want to drown our sorrows in salty, fatty comfort food. The mindfulness skills you'll learn will help you to know what to do when such thoughts pop into your mind.

Of course, besides the way you think, there are *other* factors standing in the way of eating healthy. Some factors are external, such as twenty-four-hour access to an abundance of food, including inexpensive, unhealthy food; social pressure; inadequate education about nutrition; stress; and advertising and other media. Other aspects are internal, like your personal biology, including medical conditions and mental health problems; personality; and chronic eating problems. Scientists are just at the tip of the iceberg of understanding how genetics, physiology, and hormones affect feeding behavior. In years to come, we will have a much clearer understanding of why some people have more difficulty managing their weight than others. Hopefully, this book will help stop some of the self-blame and criticism that people who struggle with their eating endure.

Unfortunately, much of what affects how you eat can't be changed. Your genetics are set. You can't eradicate fast food or your favorite treats from the face of the earth (nor would you want to!). Fortunately, thoughts are within your jurisdiction. You can do something about them.

My Background

Let me tell you a little about myself so you can understand my philosophy about food and eating. I am a clinical psychologist. Although I know a lot about food and nutrition, I am not a dietitian. Therefore, I don't tell people "what" to eat. I focus on "how." In my opinion, "how" is sometimes much more challenging than "what." You can take a textbook off the bookshelf and learn all about nutrition or obtain wonderful advice from a dietitian who creates a well-balanced meal plan for you. But *choosing* to eat healthy foods instead of comfort foods, avoiding mindless overeating, and motivating yourself to stay on track can be infinitely more difficult. Furthermore, we all have such complex and convoluted emotional relationships with food that there's no "textbook" answer for how to cope with it. The challenge intrigues me.

My focus has always been a positive, wellness approach. I'm not the food police. I don't scold people. You've seen the TV shows where the exercise guru screams in the contestant's face as she runs on a treadmill, "Just do it! You can't fail again!" This is pretty much the polar opposite of my approach. My clients have enough shame and guilt. Why add to it? I don't want them screaming at themselves inside their heads. They already do this, and it doesn't work.

Over a decade ago, I earned a doctorate in clinical psychology from the University of Denver and completed a post-doctoral fellowship at Stanford University, which is the base of my formal training. Then I began working with college students at universities and at a disordered-eating program.

Currently, I provide individual counseling, as well as write books and consult. In my clinical psychology practice, I help people work through a variety of eating issues, such as binge-eating disorder, anorexia nervosa, and bulimia. But I also help people tackle issues affecting a larger percentage of the population, such as yo-yo dieting, body-image problems, binge eating, and excess weight. Although I don't mention any names or identifying details, this information is based on my work with actual clients. Sometimes people are surprised that mindful eating can help people who overeat *and* those who undereat.

So, besides learning about mindful eating in the classroom and therapy room, I also simply mindfully observed how the people around me ate: at restaurants, in the lunchroom, and even in my own home. Like you, I love food. My mother's side of the family is Italian, so I've observed a lot of social eating and family meals since childhood. I believe we can eat all foods (yes, even treats) in a mindful way.

Here's one important note: My clients have taught me that weight issues affect people of all shapes and sizes. The pain that eating issues can cause does *not* directly correlate with weight. What's important to focus on is what your relationship with food means to *you*. Simply observing people from the outside says very little about the extent to which food issues plague their minds. And you can't tell externally how much mental anguish they are in. You can get some clues from the way someone eats—for example, if a person obsesses about every bite or camps out on the couch, munching mindlessly—but your thoughts are something only you have access to. For this reason, I never make assumptions about someone's eating habits.

Rest assured that it's possible to heal and overcome eating issues. I couldn't do my job if I didn't see people succeed. But it's not easy. I won't promise you that it will be a snap, as the fad diets do. With patience and persistence, you can make wonderful, healthy changes to your eating patterns.

How to Use This Book

For a moment, let's consider this book as a whole. When you picked up this book, you made a wonderful decision. You are about to gain many new insights and "ahas" about what's happening in your mind. There's a lot of information here, so it may take some time to absorb and think through it. Go at your own pace.

You may want to start by completing the checklist in chapter 2, which will help you identify which excuses and self-judgments you frequently use on yourself. As you read the list, you might respond *Oh, I say that* or *Yes, I think that*. Putting a check mark by that thought will direct you to the chapter that will help you. After reading the introduction, you can jump around the book if you wish. Each section doesn't hinge on the other. Focus your attention on the thoughts that ring true to you.

After the introductory chapters, the book is divided into two parts. Chapter 3 explores common excuses, or detour thoughts, that keep you stuck, while chapter 4 focuses on self-judgments, or backseat-driver thoughts, that derail your efforts. At the end of each chapter, you will see a section titled, "On Second Thought," which contains a mini mindfulness activity or a specific communication tip for thinking more mindfully. Chapter 5 is an example of how it all fits together.

If you still struggle with your eating or your thoughts after reading this book, it's important to consult a qualified, licensed mental health professional, physician, or both. Such professionals can help you unravel complex thinking patterns and identify any other issues that might stand in the way of improving your eating.

Mindless Eating vs. Mindful Eating

Before delving into the fifty excuses, I've included the definition of mindless eating and mindful eating. If you want to learn more about mindful eating, read my previous books: *Eating Mindfully*; *Eat, Drink, and Be Mindful: How to End Your Struggle with Mindless Eating and Start Savoring Food with Intention and Joy*; *50 Ways to Soothe Yourself without Food*; and *Mindful Eating 101: A Guide to Healthy Eating in College and Beyond*.

Mindless Eating Defined

Mindless eating is consuming food *without awareness*, and you may experience it in many different ways, such as:

- Eating as if in a trance or when zoned out in front of the TV, consuming food in a robot-like motion, or standing in front of the refrigerator with the door open, not really knowing what you're looking for

- Mindlessly munching while distracted (while driving the car or doing desk work)

- Eating when you aren't really hungry

- Eating in repetitive and habitual ways (eating at the same times every day or snacking during your favorite TV show, no matter what)

- Grazing on or picking at food

- Using food to comfort or soothe yourself when you are stressed, bored, or anxious

- Eating portions that are too large

- Not really tasting food

Why do we eat mindlessly, even though we know we shouldn't and have the best intentions of avoiding it? Some of this compulsion is from our automatic habits and unconscious behaviors. Eating is such a routine behavior that you can do it on autopilot or with little to no thought. It doesn't take much effort to pick up your fork. When mindless eating happens in minor ways or infrequently, it may not be a significant problem, but when you eat mindlessly on a daily basis, it can really start to cause problems with your weight and health.

Mindful Eating Defined

Generally, mindful eating is maintaining nonjudgmental, in-the-moment awareness while eating. I like to sum it up in seven words: *eat food, with purpose and on purpose*. Whenever you're about to take a bite, ask yourself whether you are doing just this. Are you intentionally and thoughtfully choosing when, where, and what you eat? Or, are you unconsciously descending into old habits? Are you choosing foods that satisfy your hunger and nourish your body rather than erase boredom or anxiety?

Following are characteristics of mindful eating:

- Mindful eating is not a diet. It's about balance rather than food restriction.

- It's not about *what* you eat; it's about *how* you eat.

- You are fully present and in the moment while eating. In other words, you notice what and how much you are eating.

- You taste and savor food, focusing on your senses.

- You tune in to your body, how it moves and feels, while you eat.

- You intimately get to know your hunger: your cravings, energy needs, and mindless-eating habits and triggers.

- You eat when you're hungry, stop when you're full.

- You eat food to fulfill physical rather than emotional hunger.

- You eat flexibly, consuming a wide range of types of food.

- You let go of old diet rules.

Getting a handle on your thinking patterns will help you cultivate mindful eating habits.

No Restricting or Starving!

As you read this book, keep this very important thing in mind: this book is not intended for you to try to restrict what you eat or starve yourself. In fact, it's quite the contrary. It's about finding balance and helping yourself learn to only eat when you're hungry. Cutting out extraneous eating (picking at and grazing on food), emotional eating, and excessive pleasure-driven eating can help you lose or manage your weight.

Outwitting Your Thoughts

Thinking is important. The way you think can help or harm your efforts to eat in a mindful, healthy way. Before you even consider changing your behavior, take a good look at how your mind may be standing in the way of change. In the first chapter, you'll learn how your thoughts may be tripping you up.

Chapter 1

Mindless Thinking =
Mindless Actions

The mind is everything. What you think, you become.
> —Buddha

Thought is the sculptor who can create the person you want to be.
> —Henry David Thoreau

Many great philosophers, writers, and spiritual teachers have come to the same conclusion: we are what we think. This idea has been around since the ancient Greeks and continues to ring true today. The nature and content of your thoughts greatly determine your behavior.

Some days it's easier to feel empowered and in charge of your eating. On calm days, your thinking is clear and rational. You choose healthy foods, don't overeat, and avoid stress-driven eating. Excuses and procrastination don't get in the way. But when you feel stressed and tired, it's difficult, sometimes impossible, to fight irrational thoughts and excuses that say it's okay to snack on junk food or mindlessly consume empty calories. It's also hard to stop beating yourself up with harsh words for not eating the way you wish you could. This is how powerful your thoughts are. The way you think can either help you cope or sabotage your efforts.

"How It Is"

We often tell ourselves a story about "how it is" and stick to these thoughts no matter what. The movie *The Upside of Anger* is a good example of the storytelling we do in our heads that convinces us that because we think it, it must be so. And our reactions are based on this belief.

In the film, the main character, Terry, played by Joan Allen, believes that her husband has left her for his secretary. Full of rage, Terry leaves angry messages on her husband's cell phone, acts out toward her daughters, and drinks too much. Believing her husband has left her, she responds to her own thoughts with intense anger, ruining her relationship with her daughters and her new boyfriend.

The end of the movie presents an unexpected twist (warning: movie spoiler to follow). Terry discovers that her husband, while walking around their property, accidentally fell to his death into a well behind their home. He didn't leave her for another woman. The "story" she had told herself was one she had invented in her head. She had acted on her perceptions and thoughts, not the truth.

We all create stories about food and the way we eat. Maybe you tell yourself, *I'm not good at healthy eating, I can't change,* or *Everyone in my family is heavy.* These thoughts and stories, even if partly true, drive the way you interact with and feel about food. Taking your thoughts as facts rather than mere perceptions can keep you locked in place.

Wishful Thinking: "Go Away" Thoughts

Why do I always have unhelpful thoughts like these? You don't think you can actually succeed long-term at losing weight, do you? You've lost some weight, but since you'll gain it back eventually anyway, why not go ahead and eat whatever you want? *As soon as I think like this, it's slip, slip, slip. I slide right back into old habits. These thoughts make me want to just give up. I keep wishing my mind would just shut up.*

—Cindy

Have you ever wished your negative thoughts about food or yourself would just go away and quit bugging you? You may feel that undesirable thoughts are totally beyond your control, which is, in some ways, true. You don't have any say over the random thoughts that pop into your mind. You might be busy at work and, all of a sudden, out of nowhere, find yourself daydreaming about someone from high school you haven't thought about in years. Or, a disturbing thought about a tragedy in the news enters your mind. You can't erase or dictate your thoughts.

Similarly, you also have little command over what you think about food. You can't erase images that pop into your mind about tasty things to eat. Nor can you magically wish away excuses that railroad you into mindless eating, like *I need another chocolate bar, because I'm so stressed out!* Like it or not, these thoughts just happen. So, when clients ask me to help them "get rid" of their thoughts, I tell them I can't really do that—exactly. What I *can* do is help them deal effectively with whatever thoughts enter their minds. When you don't let your thoughts take over, you fear them less. Consequently, they decrease over time and sometimes even fade away.

If you are human, your natural inclination is to avoid things that bother you: minimize pain, maximize pleasure. So wanting the thoughts to stop is totally understandable. But the more you try to push uncomfortable thoughts about food out of your head, the more they escalate. It's the "don't think about the elephant in the room" phenomenon. When you tell yourself not to think about an elephant, you can't think about anything else. So, if you tell yourself not to think about food, it's probably all you'll think about.

The notion of ridding yourself of uncomfortable thoughts brings to mind the movie *Eternal Sunshine of the Spotless Mind*, a science-fiction romance starring Kate Winslet and Jim Carrey. In this movie, there's a machine that can erase selected painful memories. The heroine gets her memory erased to forget a difficult breakup. While this sounds attractive, as the story unfolds, it illuminates the downside of getting rid of your memories and thoughts. Negative thoughts and feelings are uncomfortable but useful. They can deter you from making the same mistakes over and over again. They also help you to understand why you make the choices that you do. Painful or not, thoughts and memories move you forward.

Fortunately, you do have the power to choose how you *respond* to whatever positive or negative thoughts happen to pop into your mind. It doesn't sound like a grand solution, but being conscious and mindfully aware of your thoughts can take you a long way. When you take your thoughts at face value, you simply follow orders and act reflexively. So when your mind says *Eat*, you eat without question, or if your mind comes up with an excuse, you simply follow it. When you don't keep close track of your thoughts, they can run wild and take control of your decision making. They push you this way and that. When you are mindful of your thoughts, you can regard random thoughts as just that: random thoughts, not a true reflection of what you are or what you want in that moment.

Gridlock Thinking

It's clear that how you think affects the way you eat, so it's important to know how thoughts can lead you astray. Some ways of thinking may keep you stuck and lead to what I call "gridlock thinking." Consider how you feel when you get stuck in a traffic jam: frustrated, trapped, desperate to move forward? Gridlock thinking is just like this. It's a way of thinking that keeps you locked in old patterns and stuck in place. One or more of these eight factors may be behind the problem:

- **Acting on autopilot:** Like driving, you can think on autopilot. Autopilot thinking is a state of mind where you are no longer aware of your actions. You just do what's second nature to you. The mind just drives along on its own, taking you wherever it wants, sometimes to places you didn't intend to go. When your attention wanders, you lapse unconsciously back into old eating habits and excuses.

- **Having extremes of awareness:** As with the knob on a car radio, you can turn your awareness up or down. You might fret about every single thought or not "hear" any at all. Similarly, you may also obsess over every calorie or munch in a zombie-like manner.

- **Clinging to thoughts:** You have a lot of thoughts in one day. Some are true, and some are just your perceptions. It's common to react to each thought as if it were completely true and an "order" to be followed. Rather than let a thought go by, you grab it and feel the need to act on it; for example, when your mind says *Keep eating*, you continue eating without question.

- **Ruminating:** You can get trapped into thinking about the same thought over and over, unable to let it go.

- **Dwelling on the past and future:** You might dwell on the past and worry about the future a lot, when all you can really control is what's happening right now.

- **Reacting:** You have an emotional reaction to each thought. For example, you think to yourself *I'm hungry.* Your reaction to this thought can be many things: relief, happiness, guilt, fear, and so on. The secondary feeling has a lot of power over what you do next: eat, not eat, binge, and so on.

- **Avoiding:** Maybe you mentally or physically stay away from thoughts that cause you distress. Lots of feelings are intertwined with eating, some positive and some uncomfortable. You may develop habits and excuses to avoid feeling your emotions about food.

- **Judging:** Self-judgments lead to defensiveness, shame, and avoidance. Also, when your mind narrows in on a critical thought, it pushes other things out of your awareness. It's like the teacher who keeps an eye only on the "troublemaker" in the classroom. That teacher may worry about the troublemaker continuously and focus all efforts on dealing with that child. Negative, critical thoughts drain your emotional energy and often bring your efforts to a halt.

Excuses and Self-Judgments

This book focuses on excuses and self-judgments, which I call "detour thoughts" and "backseat-driver thoughts," respectively. If you struggle with your weight, these ways of thinking are probably familiar to you. Excuses and judgments can become intertwined. When you have an excuse for not eating mindfully, such as *I'm too stressed*, the mind often blows this out of proportion. It judges the excuse with thoughts like *I'm too stressed to change my eating and will likely always be fat and a failure.*

- **Detour thoughts:** These are excuses, justifications, and explanations that steer you away from taking action, hence the name. Your mind finds reasons to avoid action when it accentuates the negative rather than the positive gains that come from change. Consequently you come up with reasons to avoid or delay the anticipated discomfort or fear. "Detour" is a helpful word, because "excuse" is often associated with shame and self-blame.

22

- **Backseat-driver thoughts:** Much like how a backseat driver nitpicks about your driving, you can be critical of yourself and the way you eat. A critical, blaming inner voice can create a negative cycle: overeat, judge yourself for it, feel bad, need comfort, soothe yourself with food. And so begins the cycle again.

One of my former clients, Nina, was a thirty-six-year-old stay-at-home mom with an infant daughter and stepson, who had tried for years to lose weight with little success. Nina's biggest hurdle was getting past her backseat-driver and detour thoughts. The same thoughts popped into her brain automatically day after day and kept playing through her mind: *I'm such a failure* and *I'm terrible at losing weight*. When she had these thoughts, she felt horrible and just gave up. Her mind would come up with ways to avoid making a change. She'd think *Why bother?* and *It shouldn't be so hard*, but really, she was just afraid of confirming her inner critic's assessments: that she was lazy and a failure. The first step to overcoming these thoughts was to become more aware of how they sabotaged her day after day.

Why We Make Excuses

Excuses can also be thought of as *experiential avoidance*, which is finding ways to remain out of direct contact with a thought, sensation, emotion, or action that is distressing in some way (Hayes, Strosahl, and Wilson 1999). So, when you think *I'll start eating healthy Monday*, you may be pushing away emotions and sensations that you might not want to feel at that moment, like discomfort or fear of change. You may feel disappointment, perhaps even anger, at the idea that starting "now" would mean eating less dessert or not eating something you crave.

Let's face it. There are a lot of feelings and sensations you might like to tune out when trying to change your eating habits: shame, guilt, longing, blame, desire for treats, and so on. The more you avoid by making excuses, the less likely you are to tackle the problem. When you confront it directly, you realize you can survive all the challenging thoughts and feelings.

Keep in mind that avoidance is a coping mechanism. There's a good reason it exists. But what starts out as a coping mechanism can eventually devolve into a problem. Let's say taking an elevator makes you uncomfortable. It's not really the fear of a falling elevator that holds you back from taking it, because the probability of anything happening to the elevator is slim to none. Instead, it's what you know *will* happen that leads to finding an excuse to avoid the elevator. You will feel really anxious during the elevator ride. Deep down, you really want to take the elevator. It would be easier and faster, and require far less effort to take it. But the thought of confronting your *feelings* holds you back.

The same thing happens when you try to improve your eating habits. You want to eat more well-balanced meals and reasonable portions. That's a given. But an excuse pops up to help you avoid direct contact with the sensations, feelings, and thoughts that would occur if you did pursue your goal. You think *I'll start eating healthy tomorrow*. Perhaps you are afraid you will long for more food. Maybe you are afraid of failing. The more you lean on excuses and avoidance, the more ingrained the avoidance behavior becomes.

Let's go back to the elevator example. So you turn to your bag of mindfulness skills and try a breathing activity to calm and comfort yourself during the elevator ride, and you are successful. The next day you have a choice: succumb to the excuses your mind conjures up to avoid the elevator, or step into the elevator anyway. It's essential that you take the elevator again. The uncomfortable feelings will continue to diminish with each elevator ride.

This is why practicing mindfulness is essential. You are constantly, metaphorically speaking, choosing whether or not to step into the elevator—to confront your feelings about eating or run away from them. Do you listen to the detour thoughts or take the plunge and change your eating habits?

Why We Are Our Own Worst Critics

Self-judgments are like a dog whistle. Only you can hear your critical self-statements, but they are intense and piercing. As with using a dog whistle, you can unintentionally train yourself to fear your own thoughts and shrink away from them when you anticipate that they'll blow into your ear. If your mind says you are bad, stupid, or not worth it, why try?

You can observe the work of critical thoughts in many areas of your life. They don't just meddle with your efforts to lose weight. The same voice tells you not to call a possible romantic interest to set up a date because the person is probably not interested anyway. That same inner voice questions whether you'd be good enough to get a job promotion.

Where does this critical voice come from? It can originate in a lot of different places:

- *Other people:* Sometimes self-judgment develops from the voices of people in your life: your mother, father, best friend, or doctor, or some bully. You internalize how people around you think and what they say. It's possible to assign another person's voice to your self-critical thoughts, even if that person never said such things. Certain words, phrases, or judgments that someone said to you might get stuck in your head.

- *Personality:* Self-criticism may be part of your personality, particularly if you are someone who overanalyzes situations or ponders things for hours.

- *Media:* You may have picked up self-criticism from what you read in magazines and diet books. Diets play on self-criticism. They try to coax you to change by convincing you that you aren't good enough. Magazines and gossip columns model judgment when they nitpick about celebrities' bodies.

- *Habit:* Self-judgment might be the product of routine. Perhaps you are just accustomed to thinking through a lens of self-doubt after years of doing so. Beliefs become ingrained and can happen as automatically as getting a cup of coffee each morning or showering each night.

- *Biology:* Your biology may make you more prone to depressive thinking. If you have low serotonin levels, or characteristics of depression or other mental health issues, negative, critical thinking may be a by-product.

- *Perfectionism:* A perfectionistic person sets up an unrealistic or unobtainable standard, never achieving happiness because of the impossibility of reaching perfection. If this is your issue, back-seat-driver thoughts constantly beat you up for not reaching this unobtainable standard.

Veering Off the Path of Mindful Eating

Judgments and excuses can throw you off course. Let's look at it this way: Imagine for a moment that you just bought a new car. You are excited to show it off, so you pick up your friend, who hops in the backseat. You drive absentmindedly, laughing, talking, and paying only half attention to the road. Suddenly, you realize that this route takes you right into a traffic jam. If you were paying attention, you wouldn't have gone this way. You tell yourself *I can't stand traffic! It will make me so irritated.* So you desperately search for a detour to avoid it. Today, you don't want to feel angry. You think *I should be happy. I just bought a new car.* So you decide to backtrack a half hour out of the way to avoid the traffic jam. Your friend in the backseat notices that you're taking a detour. Leaning forward and tapping the front seat to get your attention, she starts barking insults and orders: "Stop! Turn here. How could you be so stupid for taking this route?" But it's too late.

This example is much like mindless eating. If you don't pay attention, you can drive automatically into overeating before you are really even aware of what you're doing. You get off track, because you avoid feelings you may not want to feel. Then your inner critic swoops in and starts beating you up for this decision. The result is feeling stuck.

The way you think can send you off track. Problems in awareness, reactions to your thoughts, and unquestioning belief in your thoughts, excuses, and self-judgments are at the heart of mindless thinking. In the next chapter, you'll begin to learn how mindfulness can help you cope with these troublesome ways of thinking.

Chapter 2

Road Map to Mindful Thinking

Several years ago, my mind was completely resistant to change and full of unrealistic expectations. My thinking was a huge barrier to mindful eating. Eventually, my mind-set evolved from I can't to I can.

—Shelly

Unlike other martial arts, the Japanese martial art of aikido is peaceful and doesn't include aggressive moves. Instead, aikido masters practice the art by simply getting out of the way. When a swing comes at them, they intentionally step to the side. What happens when you dodge out of the way of an opponent who lunges at you with full force? The opponent, rather than you, goes reeling out of control. In a way, mindfulness is a form of mental aikido. You skillfully get out of the way of your thoughts rather than fight against them.

Mindfulness is a unique and therapeutic way to manage your thoughts and feelings. As with aikido, you don't struggle against your thoughts. Though it sounds simple, it's fairly complex. "Mindfulness" is generally defined as intentionally drawing your awareness and attention to the present moment in a nonjudgmental and accepting way (Kabat-Zinn 1990; Tapper et al. 2009). This process includes bringing the qualities of awareness, openness, nonjudgment, acceptance, nonreactivity, and compassion to all experiences, both pleasant and unpleasant, in the present moment (Kabat-Zinn 1990). You can experience mindfulness right now as you read. It happens as you closely attend to the words on the page. Open your mind to what the words are telling you. Don't judge the information as "right" or "wrong." Just take it in.

How vs. What You Think

The very first step to being more mindful of your thoughts is to know *how* you think, which is very different from *what* you think. Thinking about your thoughts is *metacognition*, which means contemplating the "things" on your mind, like work, relationships, or your kids.

In contrast to metacognition, mindfulness is thinking about *how* you are thinking: Are you obsessing? Avoiding your thoughts? Letting your thoughts go? An example of mindfulness might be when you notice your thoughts taking the shape of a visual or audio image. Or, it might be paying attention to how long the thought lasts, how the thought evolves, and when it dissipates. When you know *how* you think, you are more in charge of your eating.

Let's look at the difference between "how" and "what" regarding a food craving. Let's say you crave chocolate. You start thinking about the type of chocolate you want: milk or dark. Then you think about the kind of candy bar you want. This is "what" you crave. The "how" would be thinking about how this craving came about. Were you stressed out? Did you see chocolate and then start to crave it? If you have PMS, do you frequently want chocolate when experiencing your symptoms? Knowing "how" your cravings pop up can be incredibly useful, because it gives you an opportunity to stay one step ahead of yourself. You can anticipate when mindless eating may happen and take extra precautions to prevent it.

Shifting into Mindful Thinking

Three ways you can think more mindfully are:

- **Be aware.** Increasing awareness, doing mindful movements and breathing exercises, observing your thoughts, and being present in the moment can help you be more conscious and watchful of your thoughts and how you eat. These activities move you into "now" rather than leave you dwelling on the past or postponing change.

- **Respond rather than react.** Mindful thinking helps you develop a new relationship to your thoughts so that you respond rather than react to them. So, when a thought demands *Eat another bite!* you mindfully consider this thought rather than automatically obey it. Also, you "hear" your excuses without necessarily acting on them.

- **Look through a mindful lens.** The mindful mind is curious and open, focusing on "now" and paying attention to each moment as it happens, in a compassionate and nonjudgmental way. As you become more mindful, you will begin to view yourself and how you relate to food through a nonjudgmental lens. This compassion will help you to be honest with yourself so you can make positive changes.

Accept Rather than Change

Most approaches tell you to just change your thoughts. If you don't like the content of your thoughts, simply change your thoughts. Don't like to think negatively about yourself?

Just think more uplifting thoughts. Delete negative thoughts; insert positive. If only it were that easy!

Unfortunately, trying to change, suppress, or ignore your thoughts sometimes doesn't work well with eating. Perhaps you've tried this approach. You tell yourself *Just don't think about that.* A study by Rachel Barnes and Stacey Tantleff-Dunn (2010) found that trying to restrict thoughts about food actually predicted binge eating, food cravings, and other eating-disorder symptoms. In other words, the more study participants tried to change or forget their thoughts about food, the worse their behavior became. The results of this study lent significant support to using a slightly different approach to dealing with food thoughts.

So, it's time to rethink the natural urge to push down your thoughts. Instead, relate to your thoughts in a new way. It may sound radical or foreign, but allow your thoughts to be what they are. Accept; don't change.

Beyond Cognitive Behavioral Therapy

Treatments for helping people manage their weight have changed over the past few years. Until recently *cognitive behavioral therapy* (CBT) has been the "answer" to negative thinking. Many therapists have been using CBT to help their clients alleviate the destructive nature of pessimistic and depressing thoughts about body and weight.

The CBT approach is pretty straightforward: if you have a distressing thought, change it to something more positive. For example, in CBT if you think *I will always fail at losing weight and then be overweight for the rest of my life*, you'd identify this as a *catastrophizing thought*. A catastrophizing thought jumps to the worst-case scenario. When you realize this, you are taught how to reframe these thoughts with more rational and realistic ones. A more realistic thought would point out that you don't "always" fail at losing weight and that you can't predict what will happen with the rest of your life. In many cases, CBT is pretty effective, because it helps you identify irrational patterns of thinking. When you identify what you are doing, you can adapt and challenge your thinking.

You probably already do a lot of CBT interventions quite naturally. For example, let's say you are having a bad day, and the thought *This day stinks* floats through your mind. You might notice yourself having a small chat with yourself or giving yourself a pep talk. Internally, you respond *Don't worry; tomorrow will be better*. Then, you stop dwelling on what a miserable day you are having and start making a list of fun things to do tomorrow. You have successfully stopped the negative thought from running wild in your brain and destroying the rest of your day.

Sometimes CBT can present a dilemma, as I have observed in my practice. For dieters, trying to suppress or change their thoughts about food doesn't always help. In fact, sometimes it makes it worse (Barnes and Tantleff-Dunn 2010). You can probably imagine why. If your mind tells you *I'm stressed out; I really want to eat something*, it's very hard to wrestle your mind away from this. Simply telling yourself not to think this thought because your thoughts are unrealistic probably won't work. Food can feel soothing at times; this isn't an irrational thought. When you try to convince yourself that it isn't comforting when it is, you create an internal conflict that is difficult to resolve. Mindfulness overlaps a lot with CBT. The two approaches work well in tandem. Mindfulness, in this example, can add to CBT, because it allows you to acknowledge that food does feel comforting at times. You don't have to dispute that fact or argue with yourself about it. But you don't have to obey the thought. You can find alternative activities and behaviors that are also comforting.

If you are familiar with evidence-based behavioral therapies, some of the activities in this book may remind you of acceptance and commitment therapy (ACT), created by Steven Hayes (Hayes, Strosahl, and Wilson 1999); dialectical behavioral therapy (DBT), by Marsha Linehan (1993); mindfulness-based stress reduction (MBSR), by Jon Kabat-Zinn (1990); and mindfulness-based cognitive therapy (MBCT), by Zindel Segal, Mark Williams, and John Teasdale (Williams et al. 2007). These treatment approaches also have strong mindfulness components. If you are interested in mindfulness, I highly recommend reading more about these therapies. New Harbinger Publications offers many books about mindfulness-based treatment approaches.

Key Points to Mindful Thinking

Let's take a moment to review and summarize important points about mindful thinking versus mindless thinking.

- Mindless thinking is automatic, often happening below your awareness.

- Mindful thinking is fully aware and open to the present moment.

- Mindful thinking is nonjudgmental and compassionate.

- Thoughts are not facts. What your thoughts tell you doesn't have to determine what you do. Consider your thoughts as suggestions rather than orders. You can turn down suggestions if you like.

- Observe your thoughts. Give yourself a gentle mental nudge each time you hear familiar excuses and judgments floating through your mind.

- Categorize rather than evaluate each thought: is it a detour thought or a backseat-driver thought?

- Welcome all thoughts, even negative ones. Don't shut them out or try to shut them up. They give you valuable information. No matter what kind of thought you have—positive, negative, or neutral—greet it with openness and curiosity. Think "mindful," not "positive."

- Mindfully redirect and refocus your thoughts. Don't let your mind run on autopilot. Choose the direction of your thoughts instead of mindlessly following the path they set out before you.

- Take a step back from your mind. Look at your thoughts as if you were watching them flash across a movie screen.

- Make your thoughts a dialogue instead of a monologue. Talk back gently. Listen and respond to your thoughts in a nonjudgmental way.

- Be patient. If you have talked to yourself in the same manner for ten years, the way you respond to your thoughts won't change overnight.

- Use mindful movements to stop obsessive thinking. Direct your attention from your thoughts to your sensations and movements.

- Mindful breathing can slow down your thoughts and bring your mind back to the present moment.

The Fifty Most Common Diet-Derailing Excuses Checklist

Place a check mark in the blank next to the thoughts you commonly think or say. Each thought corresponds to one of the fifty most common diet-derailing excuses. You will find instructions on how to respond mindfully to each thought in chapters 3 and 4.

Detour Thoughts: Excuses, Rationalizations, and Justifications (Chapter 3)

_____ *I'll start my diet tomorrow.*

_____ *I've ruined it anyway, so why not go all the way?*

_____ *I don't have time to eat healthy.*

_____ *It's okay if I eat it, because...*

_____ *I can't afford to eat healthy.*

_____ *But I want more food!*

_____ *I can't get my eating back on track.*

_____ *But I deserve this chocolate!*

_____ *I just can't resist!*

_____ *I'm stuck and can't seem to change.*

_____ *I don't want to try right now.*

_____ *I can't decide what to eat.*

_____ *I'm too tired.*

_____ *I feel too overwhelmed.*

_____ *Food is calling my name.*

_____ *I can't let it go to waste.*

_____ *It's too hard to change.*

____ I don't care.

____ But I'm not full.

____ Yes, but…

____ I'll start eating better after...

____ I hate vegetables.

____ I have PMS; I need chocolate!

____ But I don't eat that much.

____ I feel selfish when I take care of myself.

____ I have to eat out; cooking is too much work.

____ I need food for stress relief!

____ I'm afraid it won't work; nothing will change.

____ But I need something sweet!

____ I'm just too lazy.

Backseat-Driver Thoughts: Self-Judgment (Chapter 4)

____ This is awful; I've ruined it.

____ I must do it or I'm a failure.

____ I just can't say no!

____ I have no willpower.

____ I shouldn't eat that.

____ *I wish I hadn't eaten that; I feel so guilty!*

____ *If I eat that, I'm bad.*

____ *Why did I eat that?*

____ *I'm not worth the effort.*

____ *I cheated on my diet.*

____ *Why try? It won't work anyway.*

____ *I'm eating less than other people.*

____ *I'm not buying these cookies for me.*

____ *If I eat well now, I can have a cookie later.*

____ *I'm so fat.*

____ *I can't stand it.*

____ *It's my family's fault that I'm overweight.*

____ *I'll be happy when I lose weight.*

____ *I can't stop thinking about food.*

____ *I don't want eating to be a problem.*

Your Detour Thoughts and Backseat-Driver Thoughts: Use this space to include any of your own thoughts that are not listed in the checklist.

_____

_____

_____

_____

_____

_____

On Second Thought: Minding Your Thoughts

If you added any additional statements, your challenge throughout this book is to create your own mindful response. Use the information in this book to help you determine how to construct a compassionate reply.

Chapter 3

Detour Thoughts:
Excuses, Rationalizations, and Justifications

1. *I'll Start My Diet Tomorrow* Thoughts

I want to lose weight so badly. After having two kids and going back to school for my nursing degree, I put on a few extra pounds. Every morning, when I get ready to go to work and scramble to get the kids dressed for school, I vow *Today will be the day I start watching what I eat. But inevitably, by midmorning a rumbling stomach and hectic pace at the ER leave me craving something sweet and gooey. I have the best intentions to lose weight but just can't seem to get the ball rolling. Thoughts like* I just can't get started *keep me at square one.*

—Linda

Like many people, Linda has the Scarlett O'Hara approach to mindful eating: *I'll think about that tomorrow.* Who hasn't declared a plan to initiate change tomorrow, next week, or after some event happens? We often say such things simply to soothe ourselves. Having a "plan" keeps your anxiety in check even if you have no intention of carrying it out.

If you commonly say such things to yourself, pay attention to *how* and *when* you say them. Do you announce to your friends with a wink that you will start your diet tomorrow? Or, perhaps you reflexively say this to yourself the moment you pick up a high-calorie or greasy food? Maybe you make this statement on autopilot. You say "Tomorrow" without genuine feeling or without even really thinking about what it means. Sometimes you really mean it; you'll get started the next day. But, more often than not, it's a way to avoid taking action.

Take a moment right now to do a self-check. Ask yourself *If I started tomorrow, what would I expect of myself?* What pops into your mind? Does a long list of behavior changes flash before your eyes? Maybe it includes things like cutting out sweets, packing only healthy snacks, stopping stress eating, and so on. Are your expectations too high or unobtainable? When your expectations are so far from where you stand right now, you set yourself up for frustration and giving up. It's like asking someone who has only ever run a mile to run a marathon. Notice your emotional reaction to the Scarlett O'Hara mind-set versus the mindful one: *I must run a marathon tomorrow* versus *I'll focus on taking one step at a time today.* Which seems more doable and approachable?

On Second Thought: Mindful-Eating Activity

A mindful-eating activity can get you back into a present frame of mind, moving your attention from future goals to what you can realistically do right now. You don't have to do anything radically different. Start now by taking mindful bites.

1. Refocus your mind on right now, not tomorrow. When your mind tells you to wait until later, gently return your attention to the moment in the following way.

2. Take a brief moment to anchor yourself to the present. Stop imagining what you'll do tomorrow.

Focus on your immediate senses. Identify what you are smelling, tasting, hearing, and touching right now. Describe what you see in front of you.

3. Next, turn all your attention to the food you are about to eat. The food can be something you intentionally pick, like a cracker, to help you practice eating mindfully, or it can be any snack or meal about which your mind prompts you, *Eat now; diet later.*

4. Look closely. Notice what the food looks like. Name its colors and shapes. Pay attention to how it smells. Breathe in deeply. Smell the aroma.

5. Notice what's going on inside. Do you have the urge to eat—cravings? Are you experiencing any physical symptoms, such as mouth watering or stomach grumbling?

6. Pay attention to any thoughts or feelings that pop into your mind about this food. Maybe it brings up a memory or story about the last time you ate it.

7. Put a small bite in your mouth. Notice the texture: creamy, chewy? Describe what it tastes like: spicy, salty, bitter?

8. Notice yourself chewing, and any other sounds: crunching, slurping?

9. Before you swallow, draw your awareness to how the food changes in texture as you chew. Do you salivate, have the urge to swallow? Does the food melt in your mouth?

10. Pay attention to how satisfying this bite is. Has it affected your hunger level? How does your stomach feel now that it's one bite fuller?

11. Repeat and practice.

12. Don't avoid action. Take a moment to focus on taking realistic steps, no matter how small, in the present moment, like chewing slowly or shutting the bag.

2. I've Ruined It Anyway, So Why Not Go All the Way? Thoughts

I was shopping in a popular bookstore, when a woman offered me a free sample. It was a chocolate-chip, mocha shake. The tiny cup was expertly finished with a swirl of whipped cream and a little red straw. I rolled my eyes and said, "Well, there goes the diet for today." That's all it took to get me off track.

—Michelle

There's a Zen saying that goes something like this: "The stiffest tree cracks the easiest, while the willow survives by bending with the wind." Just like the stiff tree, you can easily crack when your thoughts are too rigid. *I've ruined it anyway* is the perfect example of this rigidity, or all-or-nothing thinking. This is when you think you're either perfect or a failure, fantastic or a loser. Rarely are you truly one way or the other.

Eating habits are a prime opportunity to develop an all-or-nothing mind-set. Let's go back to Michelle. She displayed rigid thinking in the bookstore. Instead of bending a little and having a sip of the mocha drink, she allowed all-or-nothing thinking to take over. Thinking *I've ruined it anyway* led her to abandon her efforts to eat well for the rest of the day.

By contrast, the mindful mind-set is characterized by openness and flexibility, responding to rigid thoughts like *There goes my diet for today* with an open mind. Mindfulness looks for what is called "the middle way," or the place between eating the whole thing or nothing. For example, you can assert *It's not completely ruined*. The best way to insulate yourself from giving up when you've taken a misstep is to practice drawing your awareness to the middle way, or the gray areas, and being flexible in your thinking. For Michelle, this would mean telling herself that a sip of mocha is not a total failure.

Consider all-or-nothing thinking from this perspective. Say you drop a tiny spot of grape juice on your favorite white sweater. If you take care of the mishap that very moment, you can salvage the sweater. If you think *Well, it's ruined anyway*, you're less likely to get the stain out before it sets. But is the sweater really ruined? It's unlikely that you would pour the rest of the glass of juice on it.

On Second Thought: Rubber-Band Thinking

Train your mind to quickly identify the first hint of all-or-nothing thinking. When it happens, mentally dust yourself off and take a deep breath. Choose to respond mindfully to rigid thoughts by using "rubber-band thinking." Rubber-band thinking is flexible and can stretch out beyond the limited categories of "always," "never," and "all or nothing." Here are a few examples:

All-or-Nothing Thinking	Rubber-Band Response
I've ruined it anyway.	*It's not too late. I always have time to turn it around.*
I'm a mindless eater.	*I am a mindful eater who eats mindlessly on occasion.*
I'll eat all of it or not a bite.	*I can have a taste; it's not going to make or break the situation.*
I was terrible.	*I generally eat well but sometimes get off track.*
I can't have one bite.	*I can eat a small portion mindfully.*
I'll eat the entire bag.	*I can eat a small portion mindfully.*

3. *I Don't Have Time to Eat Healthy* Thoughts

I run around at breakneck speed trying to get this and that done. Besides working full-time, I run my kids to soccer practice and piano lessons. Who has time to eat healthy or exercise? I barely have time to get dressed in the morning. If I don't make time, six months will go by and I'll be in exactly the same place I'm in now.

—Victoria

As a mom, wife, full-time teacher, and part-time musician, Victoria wears many hats. Whenever she thinks about eating better, her mind goes directly back to the same thought: *Who has the time?* Like many busy women, she can get ten different projects done in one day, but changing her eating habits rarely makes the top of her to-do list.

It's extremely common for busyness to elicit detour thoughts that keep us from paying attention to our eating habits, which can sometimes seem like an insurmountable obstacle to overcome. If you feel that you don't have another second to spare, try not to be too hard on yourself. You are crunched for time, and that's okay. You may find that your mind wants to defend and explain a busy schedule.

If the lack-of-time excuse sounds familiar to you, you are probably putting off eating healthier and more mindfully until a time when life will slow down. Remind yourself that you probably will never find a time that's quieter or less busy than today. As the Greek philosopher Heraclitus of Ephesus stated,

"You can never step into the same river, for new waters are always flowing onto you."

So, remember that *I don't have time* is an automatic thought. It's often a smoke screen in front of what's really going on. When you notice yourself thinking this, your mind stops right there. You probably respond *Okay, that's true* and then return to doing something else. Don't just blindly accept this thought. Think about it on a deeper level. Ask yourself *What do I really mean by "I don't have time"?*

On Second Thought: Minding Your Time and Making It Effortless

Mind your time. The good news is that mindful eating doesn't take a lot of time. Why? Because you don't have to drastically change what you eat or drive miles out of the way to go to a special grocery store. Instead, do what you already do but with more awareness. This should take no additional time.

For example, let's say you make dinner for your family each night. You think you don't have time to cook anything different from your usual meals. Instead of altering the menu, first try bringing mindfulness to what you already eat. If you eat pizza, work on eating that pizza mindfully.

Through this attentive awareness, you'll naturally change the *way* you eat and sometimes *what* you eat. At your next snack or meal, pause for just one second before eating. Ask yourself *How can I approach this meal more mindfully?*

Awareness Checklist

If you don't have time for anything else, just pay attention to these factors:

____ Are you sitting while eating?

____ Are you focusing only on your food rather than multitasking?

____ Are you paying attention to habitual behaviors, like picking at and grazing on food?

____ Are you "popping" food into your mouth or eating slowly, one bite at a time?

____ Are you truly tasting the food? Are you noticing the texture, flavor, temperature?

____ Are you staying with this bite, thinking only about this one until you finish it completely?

____ Are you gauging your level of hunger—really hungry, moderately hungry, very hungry—and eating accordingly?

____ Are you gauging your fullness while eating? With each bite, ask yourself *How full am I?*

Make it effortless. Some self-care behaviors are not optional. Somehow, in our busy lives, we find time to shower, brush our teeth, and do a number of other things that take time. It would be nice if we could think of healthy eating and exercise in this manner: that it's a given rather than an option with no emotional struggle. But the reality is that it isn't that simple. It may be helpful to link healthy behaviors to already established, routine behaviors. For example, sometimes people take their medications after brushing their teeth. Perhaps you could pack a healthy snack for work before showering each evening or go shopping for healthy foods every week after religious services.

Make the task of eating healthy as easy as possible so you don't have to exert too much effort or time. You are more likely to eat what is *convenient* than what you like (Wansink 2004). You can use this principle to your advantage. Keep healthy food in an easy-to-reach location. Place a fruit bowl on your counter in your direct sight path. Carry a healthy snack in your purse. Make grazing on and picking at food inconvenient and difficult. Hide food in the back of your cupboard, in the freezer, or on the top shelf. You will only invest time into retrieving it if you really want it. Changing the storage location of your snacks is a simple but effective trick.

4. *It's Okay If I Eat It, Because...* Thoughts

I have all sorts of compelling reasons why I can't eat mindfully now: I've had the flu, I've been dealing with a crisis at work, my child got in trouble at school, I celebrated my thirtieth birthday. The list of ways I can rationalize mindless eating could go on and on. But the reality is that when I fudge a little bit here and there, I end up feeling horrible. It typically starts out in small ways, like nibbling on an extra bite or two. The more I indulge, the more excuses I find to justify mindless eating.

—Jessica

Jessica's mind went to elaborate lengths to justify emotional eating. She called it "pretzel thinking." Her mind bent her thoughts this way and that to explain why it was "okay" to eat mindlessly. Unfortunately, many reasons for mindless eating sound perfectly rational, like *I wouldn't want it to go to waste* or *I had to eat another slice of pie, because I didn't want to offend my grandmother.*

Why do justifications and rationalizations so easily slide off the tongue? The mind can't be at rest when things don't make sense. So, when you act in ways that are contradictory to mindful eating, even though that's what you really want, the mind has to come up with an explanation or justification. It creates a mental bridge to help explain the gap.

Rationalizing includes discounting, excusing, justifying, denying, and pretending that things are different than they really are. Rationalizing statements include things like *It's okay just this one time* and *These calories don't really count.*

On Second Thought: Stop Okaying and Start Describing

1. **Respond mindfully to *It's okay, because...*** Gently acknowledge that this is likely to be a rationalization. Next, identify the self-serving purpose of the rationalization. Finish this sentence: *Rationalizing mindless eating is serving the purpose of...* For example, you might think *Rationalizing mindless eating is serving the purpose of reducing guilt* or *It may allow me to avoid making a decision by convincing me that I don't have a real choice.* Be honest about your motivation.

2. **Observe.** Instead of deeming your behavior to be right or wrong, as you do when you justify things, just describe what you want to eat—or what you ate—and why. For example, let's say your mind is trying to justify eating dessert. You think *It's okay. I have to eat it because my kids are insisting that I have dessert.* A mindful approach would simply describe what happened, without judging whether it's right or wrong. You'd tell yourself *The kids are insisting I have dessert.* Listen to what your gut tells you about this option as you merely describe your dilemma.

3. **Beware!** Your thoughts can be very sneaky. The mind can even twist being mindful into a justification for mindless eating; for example, *It's okay if I eat this cupcake to calm my nerves, because I'm eating it mindfully.* It's tricky, but important, to have a mindful mind-set, a gentle and forgiving spirit that doesn't slip into rationalizing behavior. The less judgmental you are, the more honest you will be with yourself.

5. I Can't Afford to Eat Healthy Thoughts

I have school clothes to buy for my kids, a mortgage, and too many other bills to pay. I can't afford to eat healthy. Healthy food costs so much. I don't know how I will ever turn this around, unless the government makes healthy food cheap for people like me, who are just getting by and paying their bills.

—Jennie

Being short on cash is a very real deterrent for people like Jennie who are trying to change their eating habits. It's true that gym memberships cost money. Healthy food can be more expensive than fast-food menu items. Such foods are cheaper, in part, due to federal subsidies for most grain products used to make corn syrup for sweeteners, baked goods, and other processed foods. Some parts of your financial worries are real barriers, but other times they can be another example of detour thoughts.

The flip side is that being overweight is also financially draining. The cost of being overweight is high, taking money directly out of your pocket in several ways. Obesity significantly increases health care costs (Freedman 2011). This may be in the form of higher insurance rates, more doctor's appointments, medicine for weight-related illness, and missed work without pay.

The most tangible cost is often unrelated to your bank account. Extra weight drains self-esteem and can complicate your relationships and health. Jennie's weight, for example, was literally killing her. Her weight had slowly crept up over the years to the point where she was taking medication for diabetes. Although her medication was expensive, the psychological cost was even more devastating. She wasn't able to kneel down on the floor to play with her children or walk a few blocks to the park. Jennie didn't take her kids swimming, because there was no way she would allow anyone to see her in a bathing suit. Life just wasn't as fun as it could be. *How did I let it get to be like this?* she wondered with regret. To her, the cost of healthy food and the price of being overweight were both great. Eating healthy saved her money in the long run. She bought less food overall and stopped wasting money on impulse buys.

When your mind says you don't have enough cash to change your eating habits, close your eyes and imagine that six months from now, nothing has changed. Notice what feelings and thoughts arise as you contemplate this scenario. Where do you feel discomfort? In your heart, your body, your self-esteem? Draw your attention to the emotional, physical, and psychological costs of staying stuck exactly where you are in this very moment.

Sure, you could come up with an entire list of free or low-cost ways to tackle the problem: taking walks outdoors, using coupons, not ordering so much fast food, cooking, cutting out unnecessary junk food, and so on. But at the end of the day, it isn't really about money. It's about valuing yourself and knowing how much cost you're willing to put up with.

On Second Thought: Minding the Cost

Be more mindful of how much money you spend on food. For one week, each time you buy food, whether you eat out, purchase groceries, or buy a snack at a convenience store, keep the receipt. After you eat, draw your attention to how each food purchase makes your body feel. Write about your experience on the back of the receipt. Tally up how much money you spend on healthy food and how much you spend on unhealthy options. Also factor in how much medicine costs you as well as any "diet" products you may use. Begin to think of each food purchase as a small investment in yourself, in your health and self-esteem. Respond to *I can't afford it* with *I can't afford not to eat healthy.*

6. *But I Want More Food!* Thoughts

I keep wanting more and more. It's as if I'm walking toward this invisible line that says, "Enough." I keep eating and eating to get there. Then, I turn around and realize I'm so far past the line that I can't even see it.

—Jordan

A children's book written by Laura Numeroff and illustrated by Felicia Bond, *If You Give a Mouse a Cookie* is a story that can teach a valuable lesson about the desire for more food. In the story, a little mouse asks a little boy for a cookie. Once the little boy consents to this request, the mouse asks for milk to go with the cookie. This exchange spirals into requests for clothes, a shirt, a pen, some paper, and other things. Eventually, the mouse asks for another cookie—and keeps wanting and asking for more and more.

Maybe you are like the little mouse. You keep hearing your mind say *More, please,* and one bite leads to wanting something else, continuing into a spiral. This is sometimes a problem of *desire* rather than a problem with food. We all have an endless pit of desire. Sometimes we want food. Other times we want money, homes, and cars. We want more and more.

It's difficult to truly feel contented. If you struggle with wanting more and more food, the problem you might be facing is that you are striving for a particular feeling state rather than physical contentment. You might really be telling yourself *I must feel_____.* You can fill in the blank with whatever applies to you: *full, happy, contented, pleased, pleasure,* and so on. Think about whether you might struggle with contentment in general. Advertising plagues us with the message of discontent. They use this strategy to their advantage: if you buy this product, you will be happier. This teaches us to want more, look for something better, keep desiring, and continue striving to be happy. Though being contented is unfortunately pretty undervalued, it is key to eating mindfully.

On Second Thought: Mindfully Content

1. **Center yourself.** When you hear your mind saying *Just one more bite* or *More, please* and you are physically full or feel that you should stop eating, say your name out loud several times. Repeat it in a calm, compassionate but assertive tone. Say it as if you were trying to get someone's attention. Try it right now. Notice how you feel when you hear yourself say your name out loud. It shifts your attention immediately into the present. Like having your name called when you are not paying attention, it snaps you out of a trance.

2. **Hungry for what?** When you don't feel full but your gut tells you this doesn't make sense given how much you ate, finish these sentences: *I must feel* ____. What are you insisting should happen? Compare that with *I do feel* ____. Clearly identify what emotions you are feeling right now.

3. **Practice.** Familiarize yourself with the feeling of contentment. Look for areas of contentment in all aspects of your life. Sit in a chair. Tell yourself *I'm happy with this chair just as it is. It works. I am comfortable.* This type of practice will help you to recognize when you feel contentment as you eat. After you eat, intentionally think *I feel okay.* Notice that this isn't good or bad, just all right.

7. I Can't Get My Eating Back on Track Thoughts

I can do great for days, and then suddenly I let loose a little and it's as if I've abandoned ship completely. No matter what I do, I can't seem to get back on track. I keep eating and eating.

—Mary

Mary missed her exit on the highway. She had only let her mind drift off for a moment as she hummed along to her favorite tune on the radio. She got off at the next exit. For thirty minutes, she was completely lost and had no idea how to find her way back to the main road. She became upset. Her mind kept saying *I'm wasting so much time* and *If only I had paid attention, I wouldn't be in this mess.* She pulled over to calm down, took a few deep breaths, and started again without beating herself up for where she "should" be.

It's easy to get off the healthy-eating track. If your mind wanders when you eat, you automatically shift into autopilot and old mindless-eating habits. Eating requires a mind-set of constant attentiveness.

Perhaps you've experienced this firsthand. In the morning you are motivated and energized, packing your lunch with healthy foods. In the afternoon, you say *No thank you* to a snack from the vending machines. Life is good and you are cruising along. Then suddenly, before you realize it, you're off track. You get busy and overstressed. Automatically, you grab a candy bar to soothe your nerves. This one incident of comfort eating leads to several more. You scold yourself for doing

64

well and then "falling off the wagon." The more you strive to make it happen, the less able you are to do so.

On Second Thought: Getting on Track

You exacerbate getting off track by continually comparing your past to the present. Perhaps you think *Well, yesterday I didn't overeat like this, so what's my problem?* It's longing to be where you used to be and trying to jump back to that time. Instead, accept where you are now. Tell yourself *I'll begin from where I am right here, right now.* As Mary did in the example, take a few deep breaths to calm yourself. The best way to get back on track is to be attentive and mindful *every time* you take a bite. When your thoughts drift off, return your mind, calmly and without criticism, to focusing on the process of eating.

If you've hit a plateau or are stuck, you've probably shifted into autopilot. To shift out of autopilot, shake up your everyday habits just a little. Sit in a different seat at the table. Dine in a different room. Intentionally take a different snack instead of the same old thing. Tape your favorite evening TV show and watch it in the morning instead to avoid snacking during evening TV watching.

Instead of focusing on how much you are doing, focus on the *quality*. See how you can improve, ever so slightly, what you already naturally do; for example, do the same exercises with slightly more intensity, or eat the same meal but put away all your distractions. Bring more awareness to these processes.

A Mindful Experiment. In part, you might be reluctant to start eating mindfully again right now because you are over-whelmed by the open-ended nature of the request. Your mind jumps to *I don't think I can do this forever.* Eliminate thinking gridlock by agreeing to simply do an experiment. Just this time, agree to see what will happen if you try something new. Tell yourself that you are choosing the healthier option on the menu *only as an experiment.* Your only goal is to gather information. You don't have to commit to anything else long term. Think of this as a short trial. At the end of the meal, the experiment is over. Consider your response. Was it too difficult? Okay? Better than you expected? Continue to set up small "experiments" with each meal.

8. *But I Deserve This Chocolate!* Thoughts

When I am tempted to eat something sweet, I tell myself I deserve this! If I do a "good job" at work, I buy milk-chocolate cupcakes, my favorite. I say to myself, I'm a good person, so I should have one.

—Tricia

Tricia has the Santa Claus approach to eating: she allows herself to eat something yummy depending on whether she's been "naughty" or "nice." If she cut calories at lunch, she goes all out at her next meal, ordering an appetizer *and* a main course. After all, her mind says, *I deserve it.*

Unfortunately, many of us hinge whether we eat on the value, or "goodness," of our actions rather than actual hunger. It's no surprise. We constantly reward ourselves and others with food and other things. Maybe your boss gives you a gift certificate to a nice restaurant after a job well done, or your mom cooks you a special dinner for getting all As on your report card. Maybe you make a pie for the neighbor who shoveled the snow from your driveway. "Good" behavior is frequently rewarded with food.

There is danger to attaching deservedness to food: this can turn on a dime, the flip side being that there's an assumption that at times, you are more or less worthy as a person. Sometimes you may feel as if you aren't good and therefore don't deserve to eat. Removal of food (and sometimes overeating to invoke feeling bad) is then used as a punishment.

You can turn your deservedness-based eating around by focusing on gratitude. It's easy to lose sight of the fact that if you have food to eat, you are fortunate. This statement isn't to spark guilt or make you feel bad, but to illustrate how easy it is to have a one-track mind that associates food with good and bad behavior.

On Second Thought: From Deserving to Grateful

Gratitude can turn your mind-set from using food as a reward to being more thankful for what you have. According to a 2010 review of studies, gratitude offers many health benefits. Being grateful is related to improvements in mood, self-esteem, depression, life satisfaction, ability to cope with adversity, and positive feelings (Wood, Froh, and Geraghty 2010). Here are some suggestions to help you eat with a present, grateful heart:

- Shift your mind-set away from using food to applaud your actions. If you hear yourself say I *deserve this* (or I *don't deserve it*), pause for a moment. Draw your attention to your stomach. It may help to place your hand on your stomach to direct your focus. Make a decision whether or not to eat a food based on your level of hunger or your actual desire to eat it, rather than any sense of deservedness.

- Be honest with yourself. When you notice your mind say *I deserve this food*, rephrase this to *I want it* or *I crave it*. If you have to justify eating chocolate or any other food with good behavior, it is a red flag that you aren't giving yourself enough permission to eat that particular food. Restriction frequently backfires and makes you want it more. Your mind has to come up with an elaborate reason to make it "okay." Say to yourself *I give myself permission to eat this food. I am grateful for the option to eat it if I want it.*

- When you think *I deserve*, respond with *Thank you*. Repeat *Thank you* over and over again to loosen the grip of and alter the direction of the initial thought away from deservedness.

- Tell yourself *I deserve comfort and pleasure, and there are many ways to obtain it besides eating.*

- Look at the food on your fork and express gratitude for that particular morsel. Visualize what it took for that bite to get from the garden to the table. Think of the Chinese proverb: "When eating rice, remember the one who planted it."

- If it helps you, say a little prayer or meaningful quote before you eat. You might say something like this: *I am thankful for this food, for the power it gives me, for the alertness, the stamina, and the strength.* Notice how different this sounds from *I deserve this.*

69

- Keep a gratitude journal. Write down what you are grateful for: a hot meal on a snowy day or a relative bringing a meal when you are sick. Sometimes people post notes on their social-networking pages to express gratitude.

- Practice gratitude. The more often you express gratitude, the better. At first, you may need to be intentionally grateful. Over time, with repeated awareness, your mind will automatically be thankful.

9. *I Just Can't Resist!* Thoughts

I've tried begging, pleading, and bribing myself not to snack. If I promise myself one bite, it turns into five more. When I'm totally desperate and frustrated with myself, I blow up. I yell at myself. I rant and rave, and start threatening myself with severe punishments to try to deter myself from eating: no dinner, no shopping for a month.

—Melanie

Have you ever bought Halloween candy two weeks in advance and been unable to wait to open it? You dig in and make a significant dent in the bag before Halloween even arrives. *I can't resist* thoughts are impulsive thoughts that you act on immediately. Your mind keeps saying *I want it; I can't wait!*

A series of classic studies by renowned psychologist Walter Mischel provides helpful tips for understanding impulsive thoughts. Though Mischel and his colleagues conducted these studies in the 1960s, they are still informative today (Mischel and Underwood 1974). The researchers put preschool children in a room alone with a tempting treat, a marshmallow. Then they instructed the kids that if they waited until the adult came back into the room, they could have two marshmallows instead of one. Some kids ate the marshmallow immediately after the adult left the room. Others waited patiently. Mischel wanted to know why some kids were able to wait and others couldn't.

He wondered whether some of the kids had a special innate ability to delay gratification. Instead, Mischel found that some kids simply had better coping skills, which helped them to manage their desire to eat the marshmallow. Many of these kids used distraction. When researchers watched the tapes, they saw that the kids sang to themselves, counted things in the room, or played with objects, all to keep their minds off the marshmallow.

The second successful technique for helping kids wait was to teach them to think about the marshmallow in a new way. The researcher told the children to think of the object as a cotton ball or cloud instead of a marshmallow. Kids who previously had trouble waiting were much better able to wait when they employed this technique. It cooled down their initial reaction to the treat.

On Second Thought: Mindful Waiting and Mindful Movements

Mindfully wait. You can use some of these same strategies to outsmart the detour thought *I can't resist*. As did the kids in the study, try using distraction to keep your mind busy. Mindfully shift your attention to more-affirming thoughts instead of the automatic thought *Just eat it* or *I want it now*. Call someone, do a crossword, knit, and so on. Find something to keep your hands and thoughts busy, and out of the kitchen.

You can also use a second strategy in the marshmallow studies: visual imagery. For example, imagine whipped cream to be glue or spackle. Visualize a cookie as a wooden Frisbee. Remember, this technique isn't to scare you away from treats or to instill negative thinking about food. It's to help you avoid reacting automatically to the immediate impulse to eat. As you wait for the craving to dissipate, breathe slowly. Count each breath as you inhale.

Mindfully move. Grazing and picking at food can be difficult to stop. Maybe you unconsciously pick at your plate after you have finished eating your meal. Perhaps you stand in front of the open cupboard nibbling on this or that, or sit in front of the TV mindlessly popping pretzels into your mouth.

To stop grazing:

1. Notice it. Simply observe in a nonjudgmental way *I'm picking at food.*

2. Gauge your level of awareness on a scale from 1 to 10, where 1 means being zoned out, mindlessly munching, and 10 means being 100 percent mentally present, tasting each grain of salt.

3. Be present. Zoom in on the sensations and movement of your hands. This will help to pull you out of the unconscious movement of popping food in your mouth or picking at food. Look closely at the color of the skin on your hands. Rub your fingertips together to feel the sensations. Notice their temperature. Focus on where your hands are placed. Describe how they feel on the table or your lap.

4. If you need imagery, clasp your hands together. Imagine holding a heavy paperweight in both

hands. Visualize the weight firmly pulling your hands down into your lap. Imagine straining against the weight to pull your hands up when you have the urge to take a little nibble. Remember that grazing at food is a habit and evidence that you have lapsed into autopilot behavior.

10. *I'm Stuck and Can't Seem to Change* Thoughts

I've been stuck at the same weight for six weeks. I feel as if I've found a parking spot and refuse to give it up. I can't move. I've tried everything: attempting to snack less, eat more, increase exercise, decrease exercise, eat everything in sight, eat only salad. I don't know how to get past this.

—Alexa

Sir Isaac Newton explained the concept of *inertia*, which is the natural resistance of an object to a change in motion. An object will stay at rest or in motion until an external force acts on it; for example, a ball will stay still until hit. Once the ball gets going, it takes another force, such as a hand, to stop it.

In many ways, the law of inertia also can apply to your emotional life and, particularly, to eating. You may feel like that ball. Inside you feel stagnant and unable to move forward. Your mind keeps saying *I can't change, because I'm stuck.*

The *foot-in-the-door technique* is a psychological approach that can help you get started and give you a little push. Traditionally, this technique involves getting a person to agree to a big favor by having that person okay a smaller one first. For example, if you want someone to babysit for three hours, start by asking for fifteen minutes of babysitting time, which the person probably will agree to. Once the person is hooked by this request, it's easier to obtain a greater commitment. You can use the same technique to start the process of mindful eating.

On Second Thought: Mindfully Overcome the Someday Syndrome

Use the foot-in-the-door technique. If you can't agree to the seemingly large self-request to eat mindfully today, make a much more modest request of yourself, something you know you can easily do. Choose a very small action. For example, if you are eating a bag of chips, ask yourself to skip one bite. Turn your attention to how this small request feels. Is it overwhelming? Is it "okay"? If so, make a slightly bigger request. How about two bites? Turn your attention to how this feels physically and emotionally. You can use the same technique for exercise. When your mind says *tomorrow*, make only a small request of yourself: to get your running clothes on. Your thoughts will probably say *I can do that*. Then, up the ante a little: *Just walk to the mailbox*. Once you get to the mailbox, suggest going to the end of the road. Keep going as long as you can. The foot-in-the-door technique was first described by J. L. Freedman and S. C. Fraser (1966).

Create momentum. "Move, and the way will open," according to a Zen proverb. Set up a situation where you have to move. Make it possible to feel the new sensations. Don't give yourself a choice. Remember that things in motion tend to stay in motion. For example, set a date to walk with a friend, and then leave your cell phone out of reach so you can't call to cancel. Take some unhealthy food from your cupboard and throw it away, so you don't have the opportunity to snack on it. Once you get moving, the momentum will build.

Help others. Consider the Zen saying, "When discouraged, encourage others." Join a support group, in person or online. Give encouragement to someone at work. Helping others can open your eyes to seeing your own situation in a new way.

11. *I Don't Want to Try Right Now* Thoughts

I'm constantly ordering myself around, telling myself what to eat and what not to eat. I'm so sick of being ordered around after a ten-hour shift at work that I tell myself I don't want to try right now.

—Gina

Gina has a little drill sergeant in her head who always barks orders at her, like *Change now* and *Don't eat that!* Her knee-jerk response to these thoughts is *Not now; I'm not ready yet.*

How do you persuade yourself to change your behavior when you don't feel like it? It can help to stop giving orders. Instead, be specific about what's to be done and why. Turn your attention to solid reasons why eating mindfully is important. Maybe you want to eat more mindfully to be a good role model for your kids, or perhaps you want to fit more comfortably in your clothing. If so, the trick is keeping these reasons in the forefront of your mind. The motives can be easily pushed to the back of your mind or slip out of your awareness.

On Second Thought: Give a Compelling Reason—*Because…*

Notice how you talk to yourself. Are many of your thoughts short, as if they were a queen's demands? *Don't eat that. You shouldn't snack.* Do you give commands? Rather than give yourself an order, back up your self-requests with solid reasons. Tack the word "because" onto the request. Turn your attention to why it's worth the effort. For example, if you think *Don't eat an extra slice of cake,* mindfully reword this thought as *Don't eat an extra slice of cake, because you'll feel too full if you do.* Other "because" statements that might soften your thought commands include:

- *Because you'll regret it later*

- *Because that wouldn't be eating mindfully*

- *Because you've decided to change your ways*

- *Because it's important to your health*

You may want to pick a part of your body, like your legs, focusing your attention on that area. Imagine what they would say. Why would your legs want you to pass up an extra dinner roll? *Because my knees can't take the extra weight.* Next time, choose another body part to give a compelling reason for healthy eating. Recognize that these words are not magic and will take repeated practice. Continue to focus on meaningful reasons to approach, rather than avoid, change.

Then, keep these reasons in your awareness. It may take a concerted effort to continually bring these reasons back into your mind. Use imagery. Create a detailed picture. Bring the image to mind frequently throughout the day. Make a list of reasons and post it on your refrigerator.

12. *I Can't Decide What to Eat* Thoughts

I wish it were as easy as deciding once and for all to eat mindfully. But the reality of it is that I make that decision over and over again, many times a day. It happens when I'm at the coffee shop trying to decide whether to order a fat-free, sugar-free hazelnut latte or a whipped-cream mocha. Later, there's a debate about what to eat for lunch: fast food or my packed lunch. All these details can get boring and tedious, but they merely demonstrate a stream of constant moment-to-moment decisions. No amount of planning or forethought can sidestep the fact that I must continually choose between staying on track or giving up.

—Chloe

Deciding what to eat can sometimes feel as if you're plunked in the middle of the Robert Frost poem, "The Road Not Taken." There are two paths: A and B. You stand there at the fork (no pun intended) in the road, deliberating: *Which path will I take? Do I order grilled fish or a burger?* What holds you back from boldly running down a path without hesitation? Sometimes it's fear of making the wrong decision or wariness of the unknown. At the end of the day, it may just be difficult to make any more decisions. The detour thought says *I make decisions all day long; I'm just too emotionally tapped out to make another choice!*

It would be nice if as soon as you got out of bed in the morning, you proclaimed which way you were headed: down path A or B. But it doesn't work that way. Instead of one big decision, mindful eating is made up of many small decisions that happen continuously from moment to moment. Do you order a cocktail or water? Will you eat a roll or skip it? Have butter or not? Eat another slice of pie? How big of a slice? Or, do you have a cup of fruit? Every single day, we make approximately 220 food decisions (Wansink and Sobal 2007). These choices add up quickly. It's easy to see how you could become tired. You might find yourself throwing your hands up in the air and saying, "Whatever," because you can't make another decision. This makes it easier to mindlessly revert back to the old road you know well. It may not be the road you want to take, but it's familiar. You know the potholes and hills on that road. The untaken road will bring up unfamiliar thoughts and feelings, which can be intimidating.

On Second Thought: Mindful Choices

If you have decision fatigue, create "default options." Make a list of five healthy meals and snacks that you know you like and can eat mindfully when you don't feel up to the task of making another decision. Mindfully choose these pre-set options when you are overwhelmed by decisions. Notice that this involves actively choosing, not just relying on old habits to guide the way.

Another way to create a healthy default is to only give yourself two specific options. Make sure these two choices are things you want to happen. Parents trying to obtain compliance from their kids often use this technique. If your goal is to get your kids to brush their teeth, build in a choice, which increases their compliance. Give them two options that accomplish the goal you desire: "You can either use the red toothbrush or the blue one; which would you prefer?" Giving yourself two clear, specific options can help you to feel less overwhelmed but also give you a sense of empowerment.

Remember that eating mindfully or mindlessly is a choice. Try not to be too hard on yourself. Sometimes mindless eating will happen. Consciously choosing to eat mindlessly is a better option than doing it unconsciously. In other words, telling yourself *I'm choosing to overeat* or *I'm deciding to indulge in this dessert* is more helpful than doing it on autopilot. Knowing you are doing it also gives you an opportunity to choose to stop.

13. *I'm Too Tired* Thoughts

I'm too tired to do anything different. After a full day of work, I don't have the emotional energy to try to change. I reach for the same snacks and sometimes fast food. It's just so much faster and easier.

—Anne

For Anne, being "too tired" to eat healthy is one of those "chicken and egg" dilemmas. It's difficult to say which one comes first: is she too tired and run down because of unhealthy eating, or does she choose fast food because she's exhausted? Regardless, feeling weary can very conveniently elicit detour thoughts to explain falling into old habits.

Do you frequently think *I'm too tired?* If so, take note of this. The way you talk to yourself and the words you choose dramatically affect your body and mind. Consider this example: Let's say you are angry about something. If you tell yourself *I'm so mad*, your body will probably move into gear to match this feeling. You might notice yourself clenching your fists or frowning. If you say out loud that you are tired, your behaviors will probably express this. Rub your eyes, stretch, yawn. Yawning can be contagious. Seeing someone else yawn can unconsciously lead you to yawn and feel more tired than you actually are. This is how powerfully the mere suggestion of being tired can affect your entire body.

On Second Thought: Waking Up Your Body and Mind

Your body listens to what your mind tells it. If you think *I'm too tired*, your body will act accordingly. Although you might be very drained, you can help yourself feel more energized. Imagine a ticker tape going through your mind, on which you see words that help to invigorate you: *energy, vigor, get-up-and-go, dynamic, power, vitality, vim, oomph, lively, vivacious, momentum.* Say these words out loud and notice how they give you a little jolt. Then, move in energizing ways: walk briskly, jog in place, do ten jumping jacks. This can increase your blood flow and the amount of oxygen to your brain, which may help you to think more clearly.

If you frequently think *I'm too tired*, it is likely that your expectations are set too high. For instance, you feel that you are too exhausted to cook a healthy meal. If you can't do it immediately, ask yourself what you can do now to *get ready* for when you have more energy. Buy the ingredients. Find a healthy recipe. Choose one thing you can do now to just prepare.

14. *I Feel Too Overwhelmed Thoughts*

I tell myself I can't get started right now because I'm so overwhelmed. I have so much going on: school, work, a new boyfriend. I'm juggling all these balls in the air. How can I possibly toss the act of changing my eating habits into the mix?

—Kristen

A Taoist proverb goes like this: "We cannot see our reflection in running water. It is only in still water that we can see." One step to improving your eating and exercise habits is to do nothing. Learn to be still—which is paradoxical. You probably run from place to place: get this done; get that done. You are frazzled and overwhelmed. When you overextend yourself in this way, you can't focus on what you truly need to do. Your external frenzy creates internal chaos. When I advise you to be still, I'm not talking about relaxing or doing nothing. Give yourself some downtime to tune in to your body. The stillness will help you take inventory of how you feel and help you to calm down so that you don't find the next step too overwhelming.

On Second Thought: Learn to Be Still

Purposefully and intentionally bringing moments of mental stillness and quiet into your life will help you listen to

85

what's going on in your mind. Consider how difficult it is to listen to the radio when the TV is on and people are chattering. Find a quiet place. While this can initially amplify what's going on in your head, it can also clear your mind so that taking a step forward doesn't feel so overwhelming. Remember the Zen proverb: "Sitting quiet, doing nothing, spring comes, and the grass grows by itself."

Start by being still in small ways. Turn off the radio in the car. In the shower, don't think; just be. Feel the water on your skin. Inhale the scent of soap. During this stillness, ponder your eating habits in a nonjudgmental way. When you have been still for at least five minutes, list just one small thing you would like to focus more attention on. Notice how much more clearly you can think after purposefully being still.

The Bull's-Eye Activity

Your mind can become easily distracted and overwhelmed by all of your responsibilities. To address this, draw a simple bull's-eye with three circles.

1. Start with a small circle in the middle, which is the bull's-eye. Next, draw a slightly larger ring around this. Around the medium-sized circle, draw a third circle that encloses the two smaller circles.

2. In the inner circle, specify the task you need to focus on in this very moment. This is what is happening right *now*. For example, when you eat,

your mind might want to pull your attention in a million different directions. You will be more conscious of your portion sizes if you don't multi-task while eating. Keep your focus on eating, or the bull's-eye.

3. In the medium circle, write down what you need to focus on in the short term: today, tomorrow, this week. Other things are on your mind that have high priority but don't need to be done in this very moment.

4. In the outer circle, write down the things in the big picture that are on your mind but don't need your attention until the near future. When you become overwhelmed, bring to mind the bull's-eye.

15. *Food Is Calling My Name* Thoughts

Alex, Alex! Over here! *It's the leftover carton of Chinese food in the fridge. It seems to be calling my name all night.* Eat me! Eat me! *I hear it even though I'm all the way in the bedroom. This can wake me from a dead sleep. I get up and eat it. It's as if I must answer the calling.*

—Alex

In Greek mythology, the Sirens were three partly human females who lured nearby sailors to their island with their enchanting music and voices. When the sailors got close, they shipwrecked on the rocky coast. Food can be like this. It seems to call to you, seducing you toward the kitchen. Food "calling" to you sounds like a pretty good reason to eat. Who can turn down a personal invitation?

Food "talking" to you is actually your desires and cravings coming to the forefront of your mind. Cravings come suddenly, as if a friend just called your name from another room. Hunger grows gradually, with signals from within: a growling stomach and tummy pangs. It takes time to learn to distinguish between actual hunger and cravings. Waiting a few moments before responding to cravings can help you decide whether or not it would be mindful to act on them.

On Second Thought: Responding Mindfully to the Siren Song

If you specifically think *The cupcake is calling my name* or the *Leftovers are whispering in my ear*, imagine putting this moment on hold, as if pressing the pause button. Then, take a step back from this thought. Instead of *It's calling my name*, tell yourself *I'm having the thought "It's calling my name."* Notice how this is different. The first thought expresses a "fact," while the other acknowledges, "Hey, this is just a thought. I can choose what to do with it."

Disengage from your thoughts by repeating the word "food" out loud over and over again (or whatever is calling your name, like "cupcake") for forty-five seconds. E. B. Titchener (1916) was the first person to use this exercise by having people repeat the word "milk." This is also a technique now used in acceptance and commitment therapy (Hayes, Strosahl, and Wilson 1999). After you say "cupcake" repeatedly, the word loses its symbolic meaning. It becomes just a bunch of sounds instead of bringing to mind the words a cupcake is mentally associated with, like "comfort," "icing," "creamy," "sweet," "cake." Try it right now.

Finally, turn the thought *Food is calling my name* from a monologue into a dialogue. Ask yourself *Why is this food on my mind? What prompted this craving?* Are you really hungry, or do you feel something else, like boredom, anxiety, the need for pleasure? Commit to sitting still for just one minute with that feeling. Set a timer if you need to. Notice how difficult it is not to just jump up and answer the "call" of the food. Determine if there are any other ways you can respond to the craving. If you are bored, find something productive to do. If you want to answer the craving, slowing down can help you do so mindfully. Use visual imagery. Picture a telephone ringing. You can decide to answer it or let it ring until the caller hangs up.

16. *I Can't Let It Go to Waste* Thoughts

Sometimes I feel like a human vacuum cleaner. I hate the idea of food going to waste. I tell myself that I have to eat the remaining piece of garlic bread so I don't have to throw it out. I'm always just "finishing off" the bowl. I cringe when I think about how much good food goes into the trash when there are starving people in the world!

—Molly

Molly's four-year-old son, Jack, is a picky eater. When they go out to breakfast, it's not uncommon for Jack to eat only half his breakfast. Molly finds herself eating her own meal and the rest of Jack's so it "doesn't go to waste." Other times, she eats the untouched half of her son's peanut-butter sandwich or the last few crackers instead of pitching them in the garbage. Her own mother drilled into her head that it was "bad" to waste food, and made her eat every single crumb. She didn't want to push her son to eat everything when he wasn't hungry. However, she couldn't tune out her mother's voice in her head.

But I can't let it go to waste can be a tough detour thought to outwit. It sounds reasonable and noble to put everything to good use. Remember, in general, "letting go" is difficult. Whether it's a few extra bites of food or a favorite old sweater, it's our human nature to cling to things, even if it's something we don't need. In these moments, it can be helpful to refocus on your stomach. When your mind wants to rope you into this excuse, tune in to your hunger. If you are truly full, it's okay to pass up this food. If you just can't throw it out and it isn't good for leftovers, use it for compost or animal feed.

On Second Thought: Waste or Waist?

Make a solid effort to prevent food waste. Order less. Buy and cook less than you think you will need. You can always make more. Cutting down on food waste in general will help you to feel better about it when it happens. Also, avoid buffet-style restaurants if you can. This type of restaurant tugs at the desire to get your money's worth, which is also about avoiding waste, specifically wasted money.

Simply pay closer attention to "cleanup" eating or consuming food with the intent of getting your money's worth. Ask yourself *Do I want this food to go to waste or to my waist? Will my body use these calories and nutrients, or will they be surplus?* Remind yourself that it's okay to let things go. Focus on the words, "Let it go." Imagine the extra food going into a trash bag. Now visualize carrying that bag around with all the extra food you don't let go to waste.

17. *It's Too Hard to Change* Thoughts

If I eat less at a meal, I jump on the scale. I don't know why I'm always surprised when the numbers don't plummet immediately. I get so disappointed. I think What's the use if I don't see results? *and give up. I don't see an end in sight, and just quit.*

—Megan

There's a Zen story about a young monk who wanted to achieve enlightenment. He went to his master and asked, "How long will it take me to achieve enlightenment?" The master thought and answered, "Ten years." Unsatisfied with this answer, the monk asked, "If I study really hard, when can I achieve enlightenment?" The master answered, "Then it will take twenty years." The monk asked again, "What if I work really, really, really hard?" The master responded, "Thirty years." "Why will it take longer if I put more effort into it?" the student questioned. The master replied, "When you have one eye on the goal, you only have one eye on the path."

When you are trying to lose or manage your weight, it's not uncommon to have one eye on the goal or scale. As the Zen story suggests, focusing on the outcome can slow you down significantly. It's like the question kids ask on a long trip: "Are we there yet?" Maybe you ask the same thing of mindful eating: "Have I arrived yet?" Giving up because you don't see immediate results is like going hiking down the Grand Canyon, and turning around and going home because you don't get to the bottom fast enough.

93

When you are impatient, it's hard to be mindful. You are rarely in the present moment. You are always thinking about what's coming up and worrying about being late, and have difficulty enjoying what you have or where you are right now. Perhaps you notice yourself tapping your foot while waiting in line at the grocery? Maybe you become enraged if your computer is moving too slowly. We live in a world of instant gratification, with the unfortunate downside of making us expect quick results. It's very hard to wait and trust that continued effort in each moment will bring benefits. We can all work on being more present to the moment instead of trying to hurry into the next moment.

On Second Thought: Think "Present," Not "Progress"

If you push yourself toward a weight goal and continually get disappointed, put away the scale. Hide it from yourself if you have to. Try this for at least two weeks. Notice how putting away the scale shifts your mind away from the numbers, redirecting your thoughts to what you are actually *doing* in the present moment to help yourself eat mindfully. Instead of using the scale to measure your actions, you must ask yourself other questions, like *Am I eating well today?* and *Did I do anything today that will help me lose weight?* Think "present," not "progress."

Eating mindfully right "now" instead of in the distant future offers many benefits that can't be measured by a bathroom scale. You can get these rewards right now if you focus your attention on them, things like enjoying your food, or feeling in charge or pleasantly full instead of too stuffed.

As you pick up your fork or spoon, practice checking in with yourself. When your mind starts striving for a goal, bring yourself back to the present. Ask yourself *What feels rewarding about eating mindfully right now, in this very moment?*

18. *I Don't Care* Thoughts

I ask my husband, "What do you want for dinner?" He answers, "I don't care; what do you want?" Then I say, "Oh, I don't care; you decide." When my husband says, "Chinese," lo and behold, I stubbornly refuse: "No way! How about Italian?"

—Chrissy

Many times you may profess to feel apathetic about a situation, with your detour thoughts declaring *I don't care.* You might get a sudden wave of apathy about healthy eating when you are offered something good to eat, like a gourmet cheeseburger, a hot apple pie, or a piece of fudge. Indifference seems to sweep over you. You think *I'm going to eat it, because I don't care.* But rarely are you as indifferent as you think. Buried deeply within you are stronger feelings than you may realize. How do you know? When things don't match what you really want, you erupt like a volcano. Your real feelings come spewing out.

When you think you don't care about what you eat, be careful not to assume that you are just referring to food. This thought may be another way of saying *I don't care about myself.* Sometimes we overeat as a form of self-punishment, as a way of inflicting harm and pain on ourselves rather than encountering the pain that comes from sources beyond our control.

On Second Thought: *I Do Care!*

Step 1: When you express ambivalence, do some detective work. Investigate how you feel. State clearly to yourself what you do and don't want. If you notice thoughts like *I'm eating this second chocolate-chip muffin* and *I don't care what I eat today,* list at least five things that complete this sentence: *What I do care about right now is...* Some examples might be *remaining at the same weight, living without regret, not feeling guilty later, feeling healthy,* and *eating mindfully.*

Step 2: Outline your choices clearly and concisely. Apathy is just mindlessly going along the path in front of you. Shift out of autopilot by consciously identifying three choices you can make. For example, if you think *I'm eating the cookies, because today I just don't care,* respond with *I have three options.*

Option 1: *Give up. If I am truly apathetic or don't care, I could mindlessly follow my impulses, maybe eat as many cookies as I want.*

Option 2: *Find something else. I could eat something healthier, like a banana.*

Option 3: *Eat mindfully. I could eat one or two cookies slowly and mindfully.*

Even if you pick option one, you can do so consciously and with your full awareness.

Step 3: Reaffirm that you are worth the effort. In response to the thought *I don't care*, repeat like a broken record *I do care about myself*. Think of this quote from Lao-tzu: "When I let go of what I am, I become what I might be."

19. *But I'm Not Full* Thoughts

I wish I could eat just the right amount. Instead, I eat large amounts and never feel really satisfied. I wish small bits of food filled me up, but they don't. I tell myself I'll stop when I'm full, but I never really get to "full" until it's too late and I feel sick to my stomach.

—Rachel

"I hardly ever feel full" is a common statement from people struggling with overeating. Many of my clients describe a deep emptiness in the pit of their stomachs, like a black hole. No matter how much they eat, even large portions, it doesn't seem to fill that space.

The thought *I hardly ever feel full* gets twisted into another justification for overeating that sounds perfectly reasonable. You desire a particular sensation and don't feel "okay" until you have it. Let's return to the fundamental problem with desire. When you don't get what you want, you can feel uncomfortable and unsettled. Not feeling exactly as full as you want is a difficult sensation to tolerate and feels unfair. Unfortunately, just because you *want* and strive to feel full doesn't mean that this desire is healthy and mindful. You are likely striving to have a particular feeling, like happiness, pleasure, or contentment, rather than to quiet a rumbling stomach.

If this sounds like you, your satiety cues, or perception of hunger and fullness, are probably a little off target. You may notice this when you see a list of "normal" portion sizes on the side of a box or when a nutritionist conveys them; you think *But that's so small.* Years of yo-yo dieting and being served gigantic portion sizes at restaurants can mess up your perception of fullness. Reassure yourself that you can relearn these cues. Tell yourself to aim for satiated rather than full.

On Second Thought: Accepting Hunger

Sometimes hunger is a scary feeling. It's difficult to accept being a little uncomfortable as you wait for your next meal, and endure not being as full as you want. Practice accepting this feeling. Notice that this approach is different from liking the emotion. Tell yourself *It's okay that I'm a little uncomfortable* or *C'est la vie*, French for "Such is life." When you think *Two more hours until lunch; how will I possibly make it that long?* you set yourself up for failure. Instead, think *I'll take it minute by minute, focusing on this minute and then the next.*

An Apple a Day Keeps the Grumbles Away

Mindfully eating an apple can be one tool to help you stop using *I don't feel full* as a reason to keep eating. In a 2009 study by Julie Flood-Obbagy and Barbara Rolls, subjects were given a whole apple before a meal. People who ate an entire apple prior to lunch consumed 15 percent less, compared to those who had nothing at all before the meal. In part, the apple's fiber helps you to feel fuller and more satisfied.

Another hypothesis is that eating a premeal apple can shift you into a more mindful mind-set. Consider what it's like to eat an apple or any other piece of fruit. Think about holding this piece of fruit in your hand. It's tangible, something you can put your hands around and feel its volume. An apple stimulates all of your senses with its sweetness and loud crunch. Eating an apple takes time, effort, and attention, a process that can move you from mindlessly consuming food to mindfully eating with awareness.

Try a premeal mindful-eating activity with an apple. For one week, eat an apple before each meal or at least before one meal a day.

1. At the grocery store, begin by mindfully choosing a type of apple that's pleasing to you, such as Gala (pinkish stripes on yellow skin, very sweet), Granny Smith (green and sour), Golden Delicious (golden, yellow, sweet), McIntosh (blend of red and green, sweet with a tinge of sourness), or Red Delicious (red with a very sweet taste).

2. Place the apples in a fruit bowl or put one in your purse, backpack, or briefcase. Be sure to have one in a handy and convenient place.

3. Take one apple out prior to eating a meal.

4. Hold the apple in your hand. Notice the color and shape.

5. Feel the weight pulling your hand down.

6. Before you take a bite, identify how hungry you are on a scale from 1 to 10, with 1 being extremely hungry and 10 being extremely full.

7. Listen to the crunch as you chew.

8. Notice the texture. Draw your awareness to the juice and how the texture changes as you chew.

9. Inhale the sweet smell.

10. Continue with the next bite. Describe to yourself how it tastes.

11. After you eat the apple, tune in again to your stomach. Assess again on a scale of 1 to 10 how hungry you are.

Hopefully, this activity will help you do two things: eat the rest of your meal mindfully, and tune in to hunger and fullness cues.

---

20. *Yes, but...* Thoughts

My mind always finds a way to avoid eating mindfully. I often say to myself Yes, I want to eat mindfully, but I can't right now because I'm too stressed.

—Diane

"Honey, I love you, but I can't stand it when you don't put the toilet seat down." "Honey, I want to go with you to your parents', but I think it's a bad idea." These are two examples of *yes, but* thinking. Essentially, it's a way of agreeing but then negating or disagreeing with everything that was just said.

"Yes-butting" frequently undermines an otherwise-mindful eater's thought processes and behavior. Let's say Diane wants to improve her eating habits, but every time she comes up with an idea for how to do so, she starts the yes-butting. When she tells herself *I want to stop eating mindlessly*, her mind responds with *Yes, but I don't know how, Yes, but what if I fail? Yes, but what if I don't lose any weight?* and *Yes, it would be nice, but I just can't because I'm too busy right now.*

Unfortunately, yes-butting is a very effective way of talking yourself right out of whatever goals you have, particularly efforts to change your eating habits. The mindful solution is to orient your mind to view the situation with curiosity and openness. "But" is a word that closes the mind. "And" is one that opens it.

On Second Thought: *Yes, And…*

Whenever you hear yourself say *Yes, but…*, pause briefly. Respond mindfully by rewording the same sentence to include the word "and" instead of "but." "And" shifts your mind into a position of openness without changing the content of your statement.

Let's use this example: *Yes, I want to start eating healthy now, but I have a party to go to this weekend.* Read it again with the word "and" in place of "but": *Yes, I want to start eating healthy now, and I have a party to go to this weekend.*

Notice how this subtly changes the entire tone of the statement. Using the word "and" doesn't negate the first part of the sentence. It only supports it. So, instead of shooting down the idea of eating mindfully at an approaching party, it suggests to your mind that the two ideas can coexist. You can go to the party *and* eat mindfully.

21. *I'll Start Eating Better After...* Thoughts

I'm going to Italy this summer for a vacation with my husband. It's the honeymoon we never had. My mind keeps saying Just go and enjoy. Eat whatever you want. I'm envisioning hot pizza, plates piled high with spaghetti, and dishes of gelato. My mouth waters just thinking about it. I can't go to Italy and not enjoy the food! I'll just wait until after vacation to start eating healthier foods.

—Ann

It's tempting to abandon mindful eating during holidays and other significant events in your life, like an anniversary dinner, a special date, or a vacation. While healthy eating might be a challenge in these situations, they are the perfect opportunity to eat mindfully. In fact, these are the situations in which you would want to eat mindfully, because they have the most potential for enjoyment.

Mindful eating can be a part of any special occasion. It won't ruin the fun. Instead, it may help you make sure to continue to enjoy the event. Overeating leads to short-term pleasure. Sometimes the joy and gratification only lasts a few minutes. Feeling guilty, regretful, sick, bloated, and out of control is what really can put a damper on fun.

You can gain many positive things from mindful eating. When you really taste food, you obtain much more pleasure from it. You eat less, because you really enjoy it. The moderation that comes from eating mindfully results in healthy eating.

On Second Thought: Minding New Foods

A helpful rule of thumb when you are planning for a vacation or holiday party is to take mindful bites, particularly of foods that are truly unique, extraordinary, and a once-in-a-lifetime opportunity. For example, if you are in Chicago and want to try Chicago-style pizza, detour thoughts may tempt you to delay mindful eating rather than use it in the moment when you really need it: as you eat new and exciting foods. You can still eat the pizza in a mindful way.

You can take the same approach at home. If you are going to a new restaurant or a party, eat special foods slowly and mindfully. Repeat to yourself *Less is more.* To eat mindfully, try the "shop, drop, and roll" technique.

Shop: Closely examine all your options. Shop carefully around the table or on the menu. Take your time.

Drop: Drop everything else you are thinking about. Get into a mindful mind-set before taking a bite. Draw a mental circle around you and the plate in front of you. Only focus on what you sense in this imaginary circle. Consider what the dish smells like. How would you describe the texture and presentation? (Review "On Second Thought: Mindful-Eating Activity," under the topic "1. *I'll Start My Diet Tomorrow* Thoughts," at the beginning of this chapter.)

Roll: As you take a bite, be sure to roll the food around in your mouth. Notice the flavor and change in texture as you chew. Eating in this way will help savor it. And remember that less is more.

22. *I Hate Vegetables* Thoughts

I love french fries. They are so addictive. I could eat them all day long. Unfortunately, I don't like the taste of salad and green vegetables, which are much better for me. Given the choice, I always go for fast food because of the taste.

—Molly

Molly told her husband for years that she "hated" vegetables, so she didn't cook them for dinner. She said they were boring and tasteless. One day, Molly and her husband were invited to a friend's house for dinner and were served a plate of grilled vegetables drizzled with olive oil and spices. Molly wanted to be polite, so she ate the veggies. Surprisingly, they were fantastic. All those years she had *thought* she didn't like vegetables and had refused to even try them.

It's understandable why people think they don't like healthy food. Unfortunately, our palates have become accustomed to food with off-the-charts flavors. Much of the flavor in our food doesn't normally occur in nature, but is chemically engineered, resulting in the mind's becoming leery of whole, nourishing foods. This leads to the global stereotype that all healthy foods taste like "cardboard," creating automatic thoughts like *No!* before you even try a food.

Detour thoughts may convey messages like *I don't like vegetables* or *Healthy foods taste bland* to get you to avoid trying them. It's true that whole foods do not have the razzle-dazzle of artificial, processed food, but once you've cut down on fast

108

food, your body is much more receptive and sensitive to the subtle flavors of whole, natural foods. It's like switching from whole milk to skim milk: once you adjust to skim milk, whole milk tastes too rich. When you go back to fast food, your taste buds are often overwhelmed and shocked by the amount of sugar or salt.

On Second Thought: Try It; You Might Like It

Instead of turning away from food when your mind automatically says *Stop! I don't like it*, start to work past it. Respond to this thought consciously and flexibly.

No *Way* Mind	Flexible Mind
I hate healthy foods.	*I'm not crazy about healthy foods, but I'm willing to give them a try.*
I'm addicted to junk food.	*The foods I like are created to keep me hooked on them.*
I don't like healthy food.	*I'll try not to judge them on the first bite.*
I love the taste of junk food.	*My palate will change when I start eating natural, healthy foods.*
I don't want to eat something healthy; it will be boring.	*There are many healthy options that taste good.*

Food Is Medicine

Hippocrates (460 to 370 BCE), the father of medicine, is well known for many things, including the saying "Let thy food be thy medicine and thy medicine be thy food." In a nutshell, food can be healing. The vitamins, minerals, and nutrients in foods can fight diseases and provide extraordinary, life-changing health benefits. For example, eating strawberries, blueberries, and cranberries is good for your cardiovascular health (Basu, Rhone, and Lyons 2010). There are many "functional foods" that can help your body and mind attain optimal levels of performance.

Tame the impulse to eat mindlessly, by focusing on a food's healing properties rather than just the sensory pleasure. Do some research and make a list of foods that would be beneficial to whatever health issues you may be dealing with.

Walnut Mindful-Eating Activity

Walnuts are high in omega-3, which is well known for its anti-inflammatory properties and cardiovascular benefits (Defilippis, Blaha, and Jacobson 2010). This is one example of focusing on the medicinal properties of food.

1. Put a few walnuts in your hand and then put the rest away in a cupboard, far out of reach. Look at the walnuts. Notice whether you have any judgments about walnuts. Maybe you think *Nuts have a lot of fat, so they're bad.* Perhaps you think

Walnuts aren't as bad as peanuts. Or maybe no thoughts come to mind. Concentrate on a single walnut. Tell yourself *This is good for my heart. This is helpful to my body. Food is medicine.*

2. After taking a second to look at the walnut, eat it. Listen to its crunch. Feel its texture in your mouth.

3. Notice whether you have what I call the "popcorn impulse": an automatic desire to pop a bunch into your mouth, as we often do with popcorn. This is why it's important to put the rest of the walnuts out of reach. Just notice this impulse.

4. Eat it mindfully. Look at it. Chew it slowly. Notice the taste. Do the same with each walnut. Eat them one at a time.

5. You can do the same activity with whatever healthy food you'd like to add to your diet.

23. *I Have PMS; I Need Chocolate!* Thoughts

When my period comes, like clockwork I crave dark chocolate. I become very emotional during that time of the month and drown my sorrows in fudge.

—Holly

Holly is a very mindful eater—most of the time. But, when her period hits, she caves in to her desire for chocolate. It's true that many women have intense cravings for chocolate, as well as fried, salty, and sugary foods, during their monthly cycles. It's no surprise that women with PMS seek pleasure to deal with the uncomfortable and unpleasant symptoms they experience during that time or whenever their hormones are fluctuating.

Eating a little chocolate or giving in to cravings for salt and fat in small portions isn't the end of the world, but breaking free of related detour thoughts is important in the long run. Eating chocolate or unhealthy foods for a week every month can add up, sabotaging your health over time, plus it can become a habit. Your period hits, so you automatically think *Time for chocolate.* It's so helpful to find ways to deal more effectively with cravings during that time of the month.

On Second Thought: Comfort vs. Pleasure

Rather than seek *pleasure* in food to cope with PMS and uncomfortable physical symptoms associated with your period, focus on finding *comfort*. This may come in the form of a heating pad, comfy clothes, a hot shower, bath salts, a warm cup of tea, or a prescheduled massage. Finding ways to comfort and soothe your body will serve you well in the long term.

24. *But I Don't Eat That Much* Thoughts

At work, my coworkers and clients bring in the most tempting treats. Yesterday there was warm, homemade banana bread. I just took one big hunk of it. I didn't count it on my food log. Well, to be honest, I completely forgot about it. When I really think about it, that slice probably had as many calories as my entire breakfast.

—Lisa

What did *you* eat today? Silently make a list in your head right now. When you are done, consider these questions: How long did it take you to make this list? Was it effortless, or did you have to think hard for a moment? Even in a short time span, it's easy to completely forget what you've eaten.

On occasion, my clients and readers scratch their heads in confusion. They put genuine effort into changing their eating habits, but their weight and other health-measures, like blood pressure and cholesterol level, don't seem to be shifting. Excluding medical problems, it's hard to know what's standing in the way.

In part, it may be your mind playing tricks on you. Outwitting your mind begins with being aware of every single bite. Your mind might want to try to convince you of why you shouldn't really "count" some eating. A bite of cake here and a handful of nuts there seem like nothing. Perceptually, you may not really "feel" this in your stomach. This makes it easy for your mind to downplay, discount, or even forget about it.

But each bite adds up. Even when we think we are doing a good job of tracking what we eat, we tend to significantly underestimate and underreport how much we eat (Poslusna et al. 2009; Wansink and Chandon 2006).

On Second Thought: Minding Each Bite

Use a diary, an online blog, a smartphone application, or any tool you have readily available to you to record what you eat. To reduce the problem of underreporting or "forgetting," it helps to be sure to immediately write down what you eat. Tell yourself *This bite is important.* Consider keeping a log in your purse or a spreadsheet on your computer. Use a camera phone, if you have one. A picture is worth a thousand words. Cameras help to increase the accuracy of food diaries (Six et al. 2010).

Avoid unconsciously or consciously underreporting your eating by remaining nonjudgmental. Sometimes people are reluctant to keep a tally of what they eat. They are embarrassed or ashamed of what the inner critic might say about the tally. Remember that you're not writing everything down to evaluate how "badly" you are performing. Instead, it's simply to make you more aware of how much you are eating.

Minding Nutrition

One reason you may not be eating as well as you think may be due to sneaky packaging, which can make it difficult to identify what's truly healthy and what isn't. When you pick up anything to eat that's packaged or processed, take a minute to try this activity.

1. Before you eat the food, turn its package over and read through the ingredients out loud, as if you were narrating a scene in a play. This isn't to check out the calories or obsess about the fat content. Instead, simply gauge your gut reaction to reading what's in the food. As you read, you may stumble over or skip some words. Notice whether you ask yourself *What's that?* You may find yourself zoning out a little when you read the names of unfamiliar chemicals, but this is the time to stay present.

2. After reading the entire ingredient list out loud, determine how you feel about what you are about to consume.

25. *I Feel Selfish When I Take Care of Myself* Thoughts

My kids always come first in my life. They're at the top of my priority list. Whenever I think about trying to lose weight or take care of myself, I feel guilty. My mind says, You don't have time to focus on healthy eating *or* A half hour of exercise is time you could spend with the kids, who barely see you all week. *Part of me knows this is just an excuse. The other part can't get past the "mom guilt."*

—Jessica

The safety instructions on an airplane are very specific about what you should do in an emergency: put on your own oxygen mask first, and then help the person next to you. These instructions reflect a good principle: to help others, you must take care of yourself first. Think for a moment about someone you provide care to, for example, a child, sibling, parent, pet, or neighbor. You probably know all too well what a constant juggling act it is to care for your own needs and those of someone who depends on you.

From a mindfulness perspective, the best way to care for others is to show compassion and care for yourself first. Any guilt you may feel around this issue probably comes from judging your actions to be "wrong" and focusing on what you believe you "should" do. Detour thoughts try to talk you out of eating well by convincing you that caring for yourself is a "bad" thing.

117

On Second Thought: *I Am Worthy of Self-Care*

Reframe "weight loss" or "weight management" efforts as a focus on "self-care." People naturally value the things they take care of. If you value your car, you keep it clean and get the oil changed. If you don't value it, you might allow trash to build up in it and not really care if it's dirty.

Dine rather than eat. Consider for a moment how you consume food now. Do you eat fast food straight out of the bag? Snack standing over the sink? Do you stand in front of the refrigerator picking at food? Eat in hiding? Instead, set a special place for eating at the table. Use a place mat. Ideally, set a nice plate plus silverware on a cloth napkin. Consider the message this communicates: *I am special.* Tell yourself *I care about myself and how I eat* and *I am worthy of a nice, healthy meal.*

Restore your body. An important part of self-care that many caregivers lack is adequate sleep. When you are exhausted, you are more vulnerable to such automatic thoughts as *I don't have time to eat healthy* and *There isn't enough time to sleep.* For optimal thinking, aim for seven to nine hours of sleep. This helps to keep your appetite and satiety hormones in check. Remember, sleep loss can cause your mind to become clouded, interfering with concentration and decision making. It's hard to really be in the moment when your thinking is foggy. You will probably fall into automatic patterns that take little thought or effort.

26. *I Have to Eat Out; Cooking Is Too Much Work* Thoughts

I love to cook but didn't always. Like many people, I suffered from a mild version of mageirocophobia: the fear of cooking. In my case, I was reluctant to try new recipes and, when crunched for time, felt overwhelmed at having to prepare a meal. Familiar meals like pasta and burgers were no problem. I paged wistfully through cookbooks and watched the Food Network. There was a huge gap between wanting to cook and making it happen.

—Sue

Restaurants don't do our waistlines any favors by serving huge portions and deceptively healthy-looking creations. The reality is that, in most cases, the portion size and ingredients are simply unhealthy for you. Unfortunately, the alternative, cooking, is often viewed with disdain and displeasure. A common perception is that cooking is a chore. Your mind might say *Cooking is too hard* or *Cooking is too much effort.*

The good news is that making your own meals can help you to be a more mindful eater. Cooking is an essential tool for managing your weight. It allows you to be much more in control of the portion size and quality of your food. Thankfully, it can also save you money since it's often less expensive than a restaurant.

Mindfulness can help you overcome your mental resistance to ordinary or mundane tasks like meal preparation. Think for a moment about how you wash dishes. When you become goal oriented about washing dishes, it becomes a chore or nuisance. Focused on finishing, your mind says things like *I just have to get this done* and *I should be doing something else.* When you are mindful, you appreciate each step, remaining in the moment with the movements and actions of your hands. You think *This is exactly where I need to be in this moment.*

On Second Thought: Mindful Cooking

Practice bringing mindfulness to ordinary tasks in your life, such as doing the laundry, feeding your child, or brushing your teeth. Turn your full attention to your actions. Notice the motion of your hands as you wash the dishes. Smell the soapsuds. Play with the bubbles in the sink. Once you have practiced with other activities, try introducing mindfulness into your cooking.

Choose a simple recipe and read mindfully all the way through it several times before even considering using it. Notice whether your mind sends you automatic messages like *It's too hard.* Do you try to skip to the end rather than enjoy the process? Push past this temptation by really familiarizing yourself with the instructions. Too often, you can get halfway through a recipe, only to find that you've mixed ingredients in the wrong order because you didn't take the time to read through the recipe completely. Take it one step at a time instead of trying to jump ahead.

As you start, notice your hands picking up a can. Be aware of the color of a pepper. Deeply inhale the smell of each ingredient. Place your attention on the sound of chopping. Being attentive and open to each step will help you think about cooking in a new way.

One thing that can hold you back from putting on your apron is perfectionism. Your mind might think *What if it's not good?* Try to have a sense of humor and look at new recipes as an experiment. Home-cooked meals don't have to be elaborate.

27. *I Need Food for Stress Relief!* Thoughts

As a little kid, whenever I had a bad day, my mother and I would sit down at the kitchen table and eat chocolate wafers together. This pattern followed me into adulthood. When I had a bad day at work or a disagreement with my boyfriend, my mind would automatically say I need chocolate! I turned this around by using another method of soothing myself. At first, nothing felt as good as eating. But then I retrained my brain to realize that chocolate cookies are not the only pick-me-up available.

—Cathy

For many people, comfort eating is their Achilles' heel. A bit of stress hits, and they make a beeline for something greasy, sugary, or salty. Like Cathy, we have an insatiable appetite for comfort. We seek comfort in so many ways, sometimes in healthy ways, like calling a friend, but often in destructive ways, like numbing out on drugs, alcohol, food, the Internet, and so on. Easing pain with food has become a widespread epidemic. Some foods specifically trigger the reward and pleasure areas of the brain. Unfortunately, eating is a cheap, legal, and quick way to obtain short-term comfort.

Eating comfort foods in small portions is generally not a problem. Macaroni and cheese and hot brownies are fun and taste good, but turning to comfort food as your primary source of stress relief becomes an issue that can lead to weight gain and distress.

Let's face it: the world is incredibly stressful. We all experience stress multiple times a day, maybe even every hour. The need to soothe yourself can be constant, which is especially a problem for people with little training in stress management. Your thoughts can make things worse. They try to convince you to take the easiest route possible to comfort yourself, which is often through food. If your mind excuses comfort eating because you are stressed, you are likely to get into a very destructive eating cycle.

On Second Thought: Comfort Cravings

Relieve stress. Rewire your brain to break the cognitive link between stress and comfort food. When your mind instructs you to use food to comfort and soothe yourself, mindfully acknowledge this urge. Then, agree to try an alternative way of soothing, perhaps drinking a cup of tea, wearing a comfortable pair of pj's or sweatpants, reading a favorite story, massaging yourself, writing in your journal at a coffeehouse, reading a fun novel, doing social networking, wandering around, taking an e-mail break, or calling a friend. It's often about changing your sensations in some way. Warm up your body. Cocoon yourself in something soft and snuggly. Stimulate your bored mind with a game. Repeat, repeat, repeat! Find more suggestions in my book, *50 Ways to Soothe Yourself without Food.*

Use soothing self-talk. Talk back to self-sabotaging thoughts in a calm and comforting way. If this is hard to do, imagine what you would say to a distressed child. Say things like *It will be okay*, *It's really hard*, *It's going to be all right*.

28. *I'm Afraid It Won't Work; Nothing Will Change* Thoughts

I lost fifty pounds and am terrified of regaining the weight. My weight has yo-yoed up and down so much that I'm afraid to eat anything that might add a pound. The thought of going back to the way I was makes me panic a little, and then I just freeze. I'm terrified that I can't really change. I just look at food and gain weight.

—Sam

A good-looking, single accountant, Sam desperately wants a relationship but constantly talks himself out of asking women out on dates. He has a million excuses: *I'm too busy, She's not the right girl,* or *I'm not ready to date.* But what really stands in his way, deep down, is fear. He is afraid of a lot of things: rejection, making a fool of himself, feeling like a failure at dating, and being disappointed. Why should Sam even try dating if he "knows" it won't work?

Many of my clients share this fearful attitude about mindful eating. Given their many past struggles with weight loss and changing their eating habits, they have a very deep, profound fear that nothing will change. My clients often say, "I don't believe it will get any better, so why try?" That's understandable. Focusing on the past and comparing it to now leads to fear.

When you are afraid, your body goes into fight-or-flight mode. The consequence is that you either fight against your fears or run away from them. Your body follows suit by either shutting down or revving up. If the thought of mindful eating leads to a deer-in-the-headlights feeling, consider whether fear is the real root of the problem. Reassure yourself that it's okay to be afraid. Ask yourself whether the feared event presents true, imminent danger, or is just an idea or daydream about something that could happen in the future. Fear of regaining weight that you haven't even lost is a prime example. It's the *idea* of it that creates panic. Remind yourself that this is "anticipatory" fear, rather than something that can hurt you right here in this moment, like a tiger chasing after you.

On Second Thought: Mindful Breathing

Whether you fear change or the possibility of "blowing it," slow down the physiological aspects of fear. Try mindful breathing. Mindful breathing will slow down your body and help you cope. Use this technique when you hear your mind say *Why bother?* or when it is caught up in other fear-driven thoughts.

Mindful Breathing

1. As each breath comes and goes, turn your attention to it in a nonjudgmental way. Don't try to make it go faster or slower. Just watch it.

2. Notice any thoughts that pop into your mind as you do this. Pay attention to how breaths come and go and dissolve away like smoke.

3. If your attention drifts away, that's okay. Patiently bring yourself back.

4. Notice your chest rising and falling.

5. Feel the warmth of the air as it goes in and out of your nose.

6. Repeat several times.

After doing this, how do you feel? Relaxed, more at ease?

29. *But I Need Something Sweet!* Thoughts

I made a frantic journey around the office trying to find something sweet after lunch. I needed to fill that craving, or I was going to turn from Dr. Jekyll into Mr. Hyde.

—John

John walked into his coworker's office and turned right around. Her candy jar was empty. He found another coworker and asked if she had anything sweet stashed in her desk. She handed John a bag of homemade trail mix of cereal and chocolate. Back in his office, John picked out a few pieces of chocolate and threw away the rest. Consuming the entire bag would be too much. The few bites of chocolate were all John really wanted. He felt better and was no longer distracted by his craving for something sweet.

Fighting against a craving can occasionally do more harm than good. Sometimes you have a taste for something, and it's better to respond thoughtfully to it than to try to wrestle it away or convince yourself that it isn't happening. Disputing your thoughts can cause a lot of distress and also lead you to eat many other unsatisfying snacks to try to ward off the craving.

On Second Thought: Mindfully Responding to Cravings

Here is a good way to deal with cravings:

1. Answer the craving mindfully. Don't act on your first impulse. Think it through.

2. Clearly identify the craving. What specifically do you want? Be very detailed.

3. Before you start, make a clear plan about what you will eat and how much.

4. Consider the healthiest option that would do the trick. If you crave chocolate, would a sugar-free version do? Or, perhaps hot chocolate would fill the craving but also provide protein from the milk.

5. Be fully present while you eat the craved food. Turn off the TV. Put down your book.

6. When you get what you crave, move away from the kitchen or any area where you would have the opportunity to mindlessly pick at or graze on the food.

30. *I'm Just Too Lazy* Thoughts

It's not that I don't want to change the way I eat. I'm just plain lazy.

—Paul

All you want to do when you get home is flop on the couch, get a snack, and veg out in front of the TV. You know you "should" go for a walk and don't "need" a snack. It will make you feel better to go for a stroll. But, as soon as you walk in the door, you think *Not today; I'm just too lazy.*

"Lazy" is not a description; it's a judgment and a detour thought. In a subtle way this word deems your inactivity as "bad." Let's take a look at what's behind the word "lazy." In part, the challenge is to stop judging yourself and understand why you retreat back into a corner, sometimes hiding behind a label of "laziness." Deeming yourself "too lazy" gives you an out from trying. It seems to say *Well I'm just made that way, and I can't do anything about it.*

From a mindfulness perspective, labeling yourself keeps you stuck. For example, say you think of yourself as a "late" person, because you tend to run late for appointments. You might tell people, "I'm always late," so they come to expect this behavior from you. You also come to expect yourself to be late, and consciously or unconsciously act accordingly. Begin to notice what labels you place on yourself about your eating habits. Maybe you label yourself as having a "large appetite" or being a "picky eater." Do you tell yourself *I'm just lazy?*

On Second Thought: Mindful Activity

Nip self-judgment in the bud. As soon as the word "lazy" enters your mind, become curious about your "laziness." Instead of using unproductive name-calling, which leads to self-defeating behaviors, ask yourself where your inactivity comes from. Are you a chronic comfort seeker? Are you afraid you won't be able to tolerate something unpleasant? Do you feel overwhelmed? Focus on addressing what's really paralyzing you.

After you've identified what's standing in the way emotionally, start removing the obstacles that reinforce inactivity. Hide your remote control. Take the cushions off your chair. Put comfort foods in the trash. Make grazing on snacks difficult. Store sweets where they would take a lot of work to reach.

Labeling yourself as "lazy" can spiral into many other negative self-thoughts. Use visualization to change this type of "domino thinking." Imagine a row of dominos lined up. If one gets knocked over, the rest will follow. Similarly, one judgmental thought pushes down another thought. Remember, only one domino needs to stop to prevent the rest from falling. It's the same with your thoughts. Focus on being mindful of only one thought at a time. Visualize that thought written on a domino. Imagine trying to keep this thought upright.

Chapter 4

Backseat-Driver Thoughts:
Self-Judgment

31. *This Is Awful; I've Ruined It!* Thoughts

I bought a new dress and made a solemn vow to eat only one dessert at a holiday party. Once I got to the party, my promise conveniently fell by the wayside. I couldn't resist filling up my plate with a wedge of cheesecake and a slice of pecan pie. It looked so good. Who could choose? After eating almost all of it, I suddenly remembered why I had committed myself to just one dessert. I felt stuffed and uncomfortable in my new dress. I ruined it! My first impulse was to beat myself up. How could I be so dumb to eat that much? This is awful!

—Carrie

In an old Zen story, a farmer's horse ran off, and his neighbor commented, "How unfortunate; what bad luck." The farmer responded, "Maybe." When he woke up the next day, the farmer discovered that someone had returned his horse, plus three more. His neighbor said, "That's great. What good luck." The farmer said, "Maybe." His son tried to ride one of the new horses, but it was unfamiliar with him and threw him off immediately, hurting him. The neighbor came by and said, "That's horrible. What bad luck." The farmer said, "Maybe." Sometime later, the military came by to draft all the town's young men, but because the farmer's son was hurt, they allowed him to stay at home with his family. His neighbors said, "What a blessing; how fortunate." The farmer said, "Maybe."

What if the farmer had placed a judgment on each event, as his neighbor had done? What would have happened? The farmer probably would have experienced a roller coaster of emotions: first feeling happy, then sad, then happy again, and so on. Instead, he refused to label things as good or bad, fortunate or unfortunate. He viewed each situation neutrally, allowing it to pan out as it may.

One way to prevent your thoughts and feelings from taking control and pushing you around like a leaf in a raging river is to learn how to be like the farmer. Respond neutrally to inner judgments about food, yourself, and your weight.

Stress eating, for example, is often prompted by a negative evaluation or judgment of an event: *My boss just yelled at me; how awful.* When your brain hears the word "awful" or "bad," it sends signals to the rest of your body to prepare for a "bad" event. Your body sounds the alarm and becomes flooded with cortisol, the stress hormone that prepares you for the fight-or-flight response. The same hormone triggers cravings for sugar, fats, and salt. Enter comfort food.

Now think *My boss just yelled at me* without judging. It's never pleasant to have your boss scream at you, but mentally describing the event from a more neutral stance lessens the secondary emotional and hormonal stress response.

On Second Thought: The Mindful Response

An important step to overcoming the inner critic is to be watchful of self-judgments, many of which happen on a subconscious level. While you can't control whether your mind has judgmental thoughts, you can respond with a compassionate, mindful mind-set.

Be aware of the thought. When you notice a backseat-driver thought entering your mind, give yourself a gentle nudge. For example, if your mind says *You are so bad for eating a doughnut* or *You did awful*, respond with *Oh, there's that backseat-driver thought again.* Imagine catching the thought in a butterfly net, gently capturing it to examine it closely.

Acknowledge judgment. Try not to judge yourself for having the negative thought. It's tempting to criticize yourself: *How could you have such a stupid thought?* Be matter of fact: *There's that thought again.* Or, respond with a neutral *Maybe.*

Closely investigate. It may be tempting to distract yourself with a new thought or let your mind wander away. Tell yourself *Stay with this thought.* Lean toward the thought rather than away from it.

Accept the thought as it is. This may sound radical. Tell yourself *I don't like the thought, but that's okay.*

Respond consciously. Think for a minute how you would typically respond to this particular thought. Give in to it? Ignore it?

Let the judgment go without responding to it. Allow the thought to float away as if you were watching it pass by in a parade or float away on clouds.

32. *I Must Do It or I'm a Failure* Thoughts

I must eat healthy. I tell myself eating fattening food is not even an option. But the more I tell myself that, the more I seem to resist, just like a little kid digging in her heels. You've heard the saying, "You can lead a horse to water, but you can't make him drink." I can lead myself to healthy food, but sometimes I just can't make myself eat it. I argue with myself and give myself fabulous reasons to change my diet, but I end up just being hostile toward myself.

—Mia

Several years ago, Mia vacationed in the Rockies. Her significant other coaxed her into taking a trail ride. If you've ever ridden a horse, you know that it takes skill to make horses do what you want: stand still, move over, run. Horses don't just comply. In fact, yelling and demanding will backfire. To get a horse to speed up, slow down, turn, and stop, you don't dominate it. Instead, you calmly talk to the horse in a cool and tranquil manner. The more distressed you become, the more they refuse to do what you ask. Sparky, as Mia's horse was so aptly named, would only obey when spoken to in a soft and controlled voice.

Good riding and mindful eating call for the same kind of emotional calmness and equanimity: no yelling, no distress, no urging yourself to go faster, just a calm and focused way of talking to yourself and your body.

A lot of people ride a horse or eat as if they were in the backseat of a taxi. They sit back, paying no attention, but then, all at once, lean toward the glass and beat on it. They yell at themselves after they've eaten too much. It would be helpful to be on top of the situation before the fact rather than after it's too late.

On Second Thought: The Mind Whisperer

Draw your attention to the type of words you use to talk to yourself. Are they demands? Rather than commanding that you comply, compassionately and gently invite a commitment from yourself.

Demand	Invitation
I have to eat healthy.	*I choose to eat mindfully.*
When will I be done with eating like this?	*When can I start eating mindfully?*
I must change now.	*How can I take one small step to eat mindfully?*
I don't have time to change my eating habits.	*How can I make time to eat mindfully?*

33. *I Just Can't Say No! Thoughts*

I just can't say no around food! If I really listen to my body, I hear it saying things like I don't really need another muffin, but then I find my hand reaching for it. My head says No! but my hand keeps on moving. I pick up the muffin and put it in my mouth. Before I know it, it's down the hatch. It's as if my hand had a mind of its own.

—Debbie

Do you ever feel that you've lost control over your body when you are eating? Your mind says *No, no, no; don't eat it*, and your actions say *Yes, yes, yes*. With food, this may, in part, be that your brain is overloaded. Part of you says *Yes! I want another slice of pizza*, and the other side of you says *No, I don't!* This lack of congruency sends conflicting signals to your brain about what to do. In the absence of a definite answer, the brain defaults to familiar automatic habits and patterns—old ways of eating.

Conflicting feelings leave you wide open for criticism from backseat-driver thoughts. You may hear your mind say *Can't you make a decision and stick with it?* These self-judgments serve as gridlock thinking by distracting you. They draw all your attention to what's going on inside your head so you don't tune in to your body for the answer.

On Second Thought: A Mindful No

Create congruency between your body and mind. If you genuinely want to say no to a dessert or extra helping because you aren't hungry or feel it would be too much, create what I call an "authoritative no." Ask yourself a question that brings up a definite *no* that resonates in every part of your body. For example, answer this question: is it okay to kick a small animal? You probably felt a very powerful *No!* rise up within you. Perhaps you even moved your body to emphasize how you felt, like clenching your fist. Take a moment to feel your response. This is an example of your body and mind answering in tandem.

The next time you want to say no to a dessert or treat but are conflicted, conjure up an authoritative no. As you experience that *no* in your body, in the next moment, think about your food dilemma. Use your body's shifting into the "no" position to help you refuse food. Clench your fists. Lean back. Make a face that communicates "no." Make the refusal come from deep within your lungs.

You can also use this technique to create a "powerful yes." Let's say you are being wishy-washy about eating a healthy snack. Ask yourself a question with a definite *yes* answer. Notice how your body shifts. Perhaps you nod your head or lean forward. Say that yes over and over again with emphasis. Practice this powerful yes.

34. *I Have No Willpower Thoughts*

I'm such a weakling. I have zero willpower. Don't put yummy food in front of me, because I'll make it vanish like a magician. My friend Leanne doesn't even take one bite. She has amazing willpower. I admire and envy people like her. I put them on a pedestal, as if they were superhuman. How did she get such amazing self-control? It's so frustrating. Diets tell you to "Just use your willpower" to cope with cravings. But, how do you get willpower? You can't buy it. I often wish a fairy godmother would "poof" me with this seemingly magic skill.

—Laura

Imagine that you are standing in front of a vending machine. It's 4:30 in the afternoon. Your next meal isn't for another hour and you are already starving. You scan your options. You say to yourself, *I really want chocolate.* With every fiber of your being, you want to hit the button for a candy bar. *No! I can't do it! I have to use my willpower,* you tell yourself. You wrestle with this decision and try very hard to rule your hunger with an iron fist.

Consider how different this scenario would be if you had planned ahead and brought a snack. This debate wouldn't even be happening. You'd be sitting at your desk at this moment happily munching on something you chose well in advance. In the absence of planning, you are left to choose something on the spot, which often leaves you battling with what you crave at that very moment. Planning ahead takes out the impulse factor and the need to say "no." Consider how different your choice would be if you picked a snack with a clear head instead of one clouded with hunger. Sure, you could still skip your packed snack for the vending machine. But we are creatures of comfort and more often than not go for the easiest (and most inexpensive) option.

Think about how much random eating you do every single day. Do you often feel that you are scrambling for whatever is available? What would happen if you went on vacation for a week and had no hotel reserved in advance? It's likely that you would just rent the first hotel room you found that night no matter how much it cost you. Researching and reserving a room in advance often prevents you from feeling disappointed and unsatisfied with the hotel.

People who appear to have "good willpower" often are simply well versed in laying out their meals. They take charge of their food plan instead of trying to overpower and control their body and hunger. They "can" eat a chocolate brownie when they feel like it because they've engineered it ahead of time to balance it out with other healthy foods throughout the day. Let's say a mindful eater is anticipating going out to a BBQ dinner that is high in protein. She might plan to bump up her veggie intake earlier in the day. Expect that some unscheduled eating will happen—a coworker might bring cookies to work, or your kids might ask for ice cream on a hot day. That is okay. An extra treat doesn't bother people who feel that they are in charge of their eating.

On Second Thought: Plan for Hunger Rather than Wrestle with It

Mindful eating blueprints. If you are constantly trying to summon up your inner willpower, it's likely that you are highly in need of more advanced planning. Choose one evening a week to plot out your meals to the best of your ability. Make sure it is a flexible and realistic strategy. Try not to get frustrated if it doesn't work out quite right or you have to change your plans. Experienced carpenters will tell you that even the best blueprints often need to be adapted as the house is being built. What you put on paper and what is actually built do not perfectly mirror each other. Instead, blueprints provide just enough information to give you a *vision* of the structure. Make sure to review the plan every single night before you go to bed. This gives you an opportunity to prep and get things ready the night before so you can execute the plan easily and quickly. Also review a possible plan B. This will help train your mind to be malleable about your plan.

Think "skillpower," not willpower. When you hear your mind instructing you to *Just use willpower* or criticize you for your "lack of willpower," gently remind yourself that changing the way you eat is a skill you build. Tell yourself *That's a judgment.* Unfortunately, many people mistakenly believe willpower is a personality trait or a tool you can pull out of your pocket to use when faced with tempting treats. The inability to eat in the way you want isn't a personal failure or lack of willpower. Instead, you get fatigued when you spend a lot of time and energy resisting the things you want. Consider that you are fighting a biological urge for pleasure that is encoded into your genes. Just think how many times a day we are faced with tempting things to eat. It's exhausting!

Deal with unplanned eating by cutting out ho-hum eating. People who eat well and appear to have "good willpower" are more tuned in to their bodies. They go for what they really want to eat and what would be pleasing, and skip the rest. So, it may appear that they have this amazing power to turn down sweets and such. However, it's more likely that if you followed these people around, you'd see something very different. They probably do eat sweets and good food but are really choosy about it. Maybe they only eat homemade cookies and pass up store-bought ones. Or, perhaps they look at the dessert tray and say, "No, thank you" because they love chocolate and there's no chocolate available. Instead of taking something they only sort of like, they cut out a lot of the ho-hum food options. Tune in to what you really like and pass up the rest. Ask yourself *On a scale of 1 to 10, how pleasing would this food be to me?* If it isn't an 8 or above, it won't satisfy you. You might even experience a sort of buyer's remorse. This takes some time to do, particularly if you aren't a picky eater.

Slow down knee-jerk reactions to food. People often eat with their eyes, not their stomachs. Cope with the thought *Oh, that looks good; I have to have it* by tuning in to your body. When you see a tempting treat, close your eyes for one full minute. Take away the visual image. This can help redirect your attention to your stomach. While your eyes are closed, ask yourself how hungry you are on a scale from 1 to 10. Do you just want it because it looks good or because your stomach is empty? Does erasing the visual image diminish or change the urge to eat by just a notch?

35. *I Shouldn't Eat That* Thoughts

I know what I shouldn't eat. People tend to think that people who overeat are just uneducated about nutrition. How frustrating! This couldn't be further from the truth. I've read so many diet and nutrition books that I could practically write my own. But this doesn't keep me from doing what I shouldn't do.

—Charlotte

If you are trying to improve your eating habits, you are probably constantly dealing with "shoulds" and "shouldn'ts" in your mind. Backseat-driver thoughts say things like *I shouldn't eat dessert! I must not eat late at night, I should eat an apple, I ought to stop eating junk food,* and *I must be a smaller size.* Irrational "shoulds," "oughts," and "musts" lead to expectations that often set the bar too high or radically out of line with what you really want, which can cause you a lot of unnecessary mental anguish.

Imagine, for example, that you walk into a restaurant. You look at the menu and find something you really want to eat, but your mind says *Tsk, tsk, you shouldn't be thinking about such a thing. You know you shouldn't have that.* Your brain has just set up a judgment: *If I order what I want, I'm bad. If I don't eat it, I'm good.*

"Shoulds" don't jibe with mindfulness. Expectations and "shoulds" create rules and moral judgments about your actions and self-worth. The mindful eater steps away from judgment and examines the situation from an impartial stance: no judgments, just observation. You are not a "bad" or "good" person.

On Second Thought: Mindfully Stop "Shoulding"

When you hear your mind say *I ought to, I must, I should,* or *I shouldn't,* pause for a moment. Then, respond mindfully to the statement in these ways.

- **Command vs. curious questioning:** Turn "shoulds" into questions. For example, instead of thinking *I shouldn't eat that cheesecake,* ask yourself *Would I be eating mindfully if I ate the cheesecake?* Notice how this shifts from a judgment to an inquisitive, neutral stance.

- **Must vs. desire:** State the "should" as a desire rather than a rule to follow. Turn *I must lose weight* into *I'd like to lose weight.* This approach redirects you from thinking about your behavior as "right" or "wrong," which is, again, a judgment.

- **Add-in vs. subtract mentality:** Try to stop working from a subtraction mind-set. This is thinking about what you can *cut out* of your diet. This type of thinking causes cravings and longings for food. It also leads to feeling deprived. Instead, start from the mind-set of what you can *add in* to your day. Imagine starting with an empty plate to be filled up with good foods. Build *up* your diet instead of taking food *away*.

- **Hunger vs. rules:** Work on using hunger-based cues to decide what to eat instead of "should" statements. This can be a major shift in thinking. You may be more familiar with diet rules that dictate what you "ought" to do. Initially, it can be very scary to follow your instincts instead of concrete rules. Before you eat, check in with your stomach. Ask yourself how hungry you are on a scale of 1 to 10. Watch out for old diet rules that pop into your head. For example, instead of thinking *I shouldn't eat a snack after eight o'clock*, ask yourself *How hungry am I right now?* Turn your locus of control inward. Remember that following rigid rules is different from giving yourself some flexible boundaries and guidelines.

36. *I Wish I Hadn't Eaten That; I Feel So Guilty!* Thoughts

My mom never touched a croissant, because she believed it was too fattening. If I eat one, it triggers intense food guilt. I can hear my mother's voice in my head warning me about the evils of buttery, flaky bread, but I can't help it. I love it: bite, yum, ah. Then, the guilt ensues. I keep rehashing it in my mind, trying to make the guilt go away.

—Lizzy

My clients pose this question each and every day: "What do I do when I feel guilty after eating? How can I make it stop?" Guilt can hang around for a mildly annoying few minutes or completely ruin your entire week. Why does food guilt cause such turmoil?

The desire to squash food guilt is quite natural. When my clients bring up this wish, I gently remind them of the saying, "Don't kill the messenger," a phrase that dates back to ancient Greece. Prior to phones, faxes, and cars, messages, particularly during times of war, were delivered in person. Unfortunately, when delivering bad news, the messenger sometimes would be executed simply for bearing such information. Your feelings and thoughts, no matter how negative, are messengers delivering important communication to you.

Guilt is your body sending you a distress message, such as *You ate too much.* This is good information to have. Try to take this as a useful message instead of twisting and turning it into guilt and shame. For example, this message can help you gauge how much to eat in the future.

Remember that guilt will pass if you give it time. While you wait, your job is not to make it worse. Judging yourself is like throwing gasoline on a fire. You can feed these thoughts or allow the fire to slowly burn out. The danger is that when you fuel guilt, you feel bad and then need comfort, putting you at a high risk for emotional eating.

Suffering comes from wrestling with your mind and striving not to feel. It's like pushing really hard against the door to keep something out. If you've experienced food guilt, you know that the guilty feelings are sometimes much worse than the actual physical sensation of overeating.

On Second Thought: Welcome the Guilt Messenger

Instead of trying to fight off the guilt, welcome it in. This may sound radical or foreign to you. When you have a thought you don't want, remind yourself *Don't kill the messenger.* If you feel guilty, try not to wiggle out of that feeling or wish it away. You might find yourself making deals with yourself to make the guilt stop: *I won't eat tonight so that I don't have to feel guilty.*

Gently acknowledge your feelings, and compassionately and with an open curiosity, ask yourself these questions:

- *What is the thought messenger saying?*

- *What is it trying to teach me?*

- *What can I learn from this message?*

- *Why am I trying to avoid this message?*

37. *If I Eat That, I'm Bad Thoughts*

When I'm about to eat something yummy, I always feel that I'm doing something bad, really bad. It's weird because it's not as if I've committed a crime, but I feel the same kind of guilt. I eat dessert equals I'm bad. I eat fruit equals I'm good.

—Faye

Health magazines frequently feature "good" and "bad" foods. As a psychologist, I can't help but cringe when reading articles that bash foods and describe them in evil terms. Using the terms "bad" and "good" to evaluate foods sets people up for a moral battle over what they consume. It turns into this: *If I eat bad foods, I'm bad*, which inevitably ends in guilt. If you want to conquer a complicated relationship with food, a helpful step is to stop demonizing foods. Then, in turn, don't judge yourself as "good" or "bad" for what you eat.

It's true that some foods are significantly healthier and less toxic than others, but beware of how easily this is twisted into a judgment. To avoid the "good" and "bad" debate, one of my former clients asked herself this question: *If I ate this very food every day for the next ten years, would it harm me or help me?*

On Second Thought: Mindful Words

To ease guilt out of the eating equation, closely draw your awareness to your thoughts. Notice the words you use. If they are evaluative—"good," "bad," "terrible," "great"—aim for something more neutral. Instead, there are "more skillful" and "less skillful" ways of acting. Stick with "healthier" and "less healthy" instead of "good" and "bad" food.

It can help to *categorize* the content rather than *evaluate* it as "good" or "bad." When you classify something, begin the sentence with the word "There's." For example, if you think *I believe*, then respond *There's a thought*.

- If you think *This is awful!* respond *There's a judgment*.

- *If you have a rising feeling of guilt*, respond *There's an emotion*.

- *If you notice that your hand is warm*, respond *There's a sensation*.

Try this today. Engage in classifying whatever arises in your mind. Here are some categories: emotions, thoughts, sensations, cravings, judgments, excuses, impulses, memories.

38. *Why Did I Eat That?* Thoughts

Oh my, why did I have all those holiday desserts? A can-noli, a decorated sugar cookie, a piece of pumpkin pie—I feel so guilty! I just keep replaying in my head all the things I ate.

—Katelyn

Have you ever had this thought? *I just want to turn my mind off!* Your thoughts are like a song stuck on repeat. Sometimes you can't even sleep, because your mind won't shut down. You can let most thoughts slide by you, but for some reason, when your thoughts are of food guilt, your mind races and just won't let them go.

Let's say you can't let go of the thought *I feel so guilty after I eat.* You may be stuck on this thought because your mind tries to "solve" this problem: *What should I do to make this better?* Unfortunately, this is where you get stuck in gridlock thinking. There's no solution or way to undo eating what you ate.

Use mindfulness skills to help you cope with how miserable you feel after overeating. This is not intended to make you forget what you've done, but obsessing about what you ate will only serve to intensify your emotional distress. The more you think about it, the more upset you become, which often leads to comfort eating.

On Second Thought: Unregrettable Moments

When you hear your mind focusing on guilt, choose to respond with "regret," a more neutral word. Because guilt is based on shame, "regret" shifts your focus off judgment and onto the problem or consequence. When your mind wants to rehash everything you regret eating, try to stay in this moment, the present moment, instead of letting your mind drift into the past.

Focus on what you can do to make this moment unregrettable. It may be tempting to get into black-and-white thinking with thoughts like *Well, I've ruined it anyway.* Instead, remember that you can't change the past, but you can be present and mindful in this very moment. Sometimes the simple passing of time is the only thing that makes regret lessen. As you wait, work on forgiving yourself. Remind yourself *This, too, shall pass. This feeling will dissipate over time.*

Make It a Guilt-Free Moment

Create a list of things you can do that are guilt free and help you disengage from your thoughts. Some examples are:

- Turning down the lights

- Taking a breather

- Saying a prayer of forgiveness

- Saying a kind word to yourself or someone else

- Doing something nice for a friend

- Intentionally taking a mindful bite if you are eating

39. *I'm Not Worth the Effort* Thoughts

Why should I put the effort into taking care of myself? I don't feel worth it. The bigger question is how do I remember that I'm valuable and worthy of care in the middle of a craving for chocolate, birthday cake, onion rings, and the like?

—Brooke

Brooke was a participant in one of my mindful-eating workshops. Each week, she came to the mindful-eating group and confessed her mindless-eating slips. The group expressed concern and asked Brooke what led her to knowingly self-sabotage over and over again. "I'm not worth it," she responded.

Her backseat-driver thoughts convinced her that she wasn't a valued member of society. In her mind, it didn't matter if she got healthier or not. *What could I possibly add to the world?* she thought. It was easy to see why Brooke struggled with self-worth. She had been abused as a teen and divorced twice, and struggled with chronic overeating. She had lost and regained over a hundred pounds in her life. Food didn't disappoint her, whereas people did. Her feelings of self-worth had slowly drained away over the years.

A woman in the group profoundly changed Brooke's outlook. After one of Brooke's confessions and self-devaluations, the woman reached into her purse, delving her hand deeply into its recesses and eventually pulling out a five-dollar bill.

The money had been stuffed in carelessly and had become quite beaten and torn.

The woman said, "It's easy to get lost and abused in the bottom of my purse. There's a lot of garbage in there. No matter how much this money has been beaten up, it still holds value. It's still worth the same amount."

The lesson is that you have value no matter what has happened to you. This value is fixed, unchanging. Too often, people try to hinge their self-worth on things that do change, like income, relationships, and weight. When people challenge their own worth, they tend to give up on themselves. They feel like a piece of costume jewelry parading around as the real thing. *Why polish it if it's fake?* they ask.

For Brooke and all mindful eaters, self-acceptance is important and the exact opposite of evaluating your personal worth. Self-acceptance deems you to be okay just as you are. This is a tough notion for overeaters to believe. Brooke was a good example of this. Tallying up her "value" interfered with her ability to take care of herself. Brooke turned this around by working on self-acceptance.

On Second Thought: Loving-Kindness Meditation

Repeat a loving-kindness meditation when you don't feel worth the effort: *May I take care of myself; may I be healthy; may I be free from self-judgment; may I eat mindfully.* You can alter it as you see fit. The traditional form of this meditation is to first direct this kindness toward yourself and then to direct it to others, as follows:

1. Yourself (*May I take care of myself…*)

2. A good friend (*May my friend take care of herself…*)

3. A "neutral" person (like an acquaintance or neighbor)

4. A difficult person

5. All four of the previous people equally

6. Gradually, the entire universe

40. *I Cheated on My Diet* Thoughts

I didn't touch the cinnamon coffee cake. I was a saint. When I cheat on my diet, I feel as if I were actually cheating on my significant other—so guilty!

—Kelly

Have you ever used words like "cheated" and "stole a bite" to describe your eating, or said to yourself *I have to pay* for eating high-calorie snacks? Backseat-driver thoughts play on guilt and the notion of *culpability*, which means the extent you are to blame for an action. In legal forums, the word describes how much someone is at fault for committing a crime, which is important because it affects the severity of the person's punishment.

Perhaps you feel as if you are on trial when you eat, as if a judge and jury are reviewing the facts to determine if you are to blame for overeating. If you are guilty, maybe you sentence yourself to some punishment, perhaps no dinner after an overeating episode.

Instead of focusing on culpability, aim for accountability to help keep you on track. *Accountability* is nonjudgmentally drawing your awareness to your behavior. You may already do this with other behaviors, such as keeping your checkbook or punching a time card. These practices aren't to judge your behavior but to make you aware of exactly how much you spend and whether you are working the expected number of hours.

On Second Thought:
Accountability, Not Culpability

Step away from self-judgment by drawing your attention to accountability rather than finger-pointing.

- Reframing "cheating" as "mindless eating" helps remove judgment.

- Your clothing can help to keep you accountable and aware. Weight gain and loss often happens slowly and below your awareness. Clothing is one of your best tools to help you notice any changes in your body that can alert you to the need to pay closer attention to your eating. Choose a pair of pants that you wear frequently. Put them on once a week to help you gain a better sense of where you are.

- Identify an accountability friend. Rather than confess your "food sins," just state in a matter-of-fact, nonjudgmental way what you regret.

- Create a journal, or a blog (with a pseudonym). Blogs are a wonderful way to help keep you accountable. You'll find that your online supporters will notice your absence, give you new ideas, and provide encouragement.

- Involve loved ones in a plan to keep you accountable. For example, commit to avoiding eating mindlessly in front of your kids so you can be a healthy role model. Or, join with your spouse in agreeing not to buy unhealthy snacks.

- Take a mindful moment at the end of each day to check in with yourself about your successes and challenges of the day.

41. *Why Try? It Won't Work Anyway* Thoughts

Why bother? I try and always fail. Although on the out-side, I look as if I'm trying, on the inside I don't believe even for a moment that it'll work.

—Emmy

How do you feel when you read Emmy's statement? Hopeless, unmotivated? *It won't work anyway* thoughts are an example of a *self-fulfilling prophecy*, which is a prediction that, directly or indirectly, results in the feared outcome.

Forms of the word "prophecy" have existed from the time of ancient Greece. People from antiquity wanted to know what would happen in the future, so they consulted oracles, astrologers, and fortune-tellers. In fact, when the Buddha was born, around 600 BCE, his parents, the king and queen of an area that's now part of India or Nepal, consulted a fortune-teller to predict their son's future profession. The fortune-teller indicated that he would either be the next king or a spiritual leader, a prediction that greatly affected the parents' actions. From the time the Buddha was born, they tried steering him toward becoming the next king, giving him a grand lifestyle in hopes he would live out that part of the prophecy.

Obviously, he didn't live out that prophecy. He made a decision based on his life circumstances in the moment rather than on his parents' interpretation of the prediction during his infancy.

Self-fulfilling prophecies can greatly affect how you eat. If you think you'll fail, your behavior probably will unconsciously

163

or consciously make it happen. If you think you won't be able to turn around your eating, you probably will act in ways that lead you there. You might self-sabotage by snacking on unhealthy food or mindlessly eating when you aren't hungry.

Mindfulness allows you to see things as they are in this moment, not as you think they will be in the future or how they were in the past. The thought *It won't work* urges you to jump ahead and try to predict the future instead of staying in the present moment.

On Second Thought: In the Now

Too often, we are like the ancient Greeks and the Buddha's parents, attempting to predict the future. Return your mind to the moment by focusing only on what's happening right now. Keep your mind anchored to the present moment: this day, this minute, this second. When your mind tries to push you ahead with statements like *Why try? I'll regain the weight anyway* or *I should be thinner by my sister's wedding date*, return to the moment. Try the following imagery.

The Balance Beam

Imagine walking on a balance beam. Visualize looking down at your feet to try to stay centered. Focus only on keeping your feet on the balance beam. When your mind wants to pull you into reviewing your eating or worrying about the future, imagine your foot veering off the balance beam. If you continue moving in that direction, you'll fall. Imagine replacing the foot, positioning yourself again to only focus on your feet, and moving forward. Keep your mind centered on the present.

Small Victories

For one week make a list of at least five small victories you have each day. Small victories are events that are happening now that lead you toward mindful eating. They can be as simple as taking the stairs instead of the elevator, or passing up an extra cookie. Unfortunately, we often focus on our mistakes. Train your mind to notice and be attentive to the healthy steps you are taking.

42. *I'm Eating Less than Other People* Thoughts

I compare myself to everyone around me almost on a daily basis. I evaluate whether I'm thinner, prettier, or more successful. I often walk away feeling like a failure and not good enough. My brain constantly sizes up what others eat compared to what I eat. Are they eating more, less, healthier, or more-fattening foods?

—Betsy

I can usually detect when my clients are struggling with competitiveness. They notice what the people around them eat for dinner and keep tabs on what a significant other has for a snack. They talk about how much their friends weigh and notice when a coworker loses or gains weight.

It's hard not to do some comparing. We all want to be within the "norm." The kind of comparing I'm talking about takes place with a spirit of judgment. You deem yourself to be a "better" or "worse" eater than someone else. You might look at weight loss as a competition or seek to equal someone else's success instead of to be healthier.

Inevitably, comparing yourself to others doesn't work in your favor and is heavily influenced by context. Say you are eating dinner with a group of sumo wrestlers. How would you judge your eating when you compare it to that of the rest of the group? Now, compare your eating to that of runway models. The point is that the person to whom you compare yourself dramatically influences how you will feel.

Some comparing may happen on an unconscious level, automatically. It happens so effortlessly that you don't even realize you're sizing someone up. At other times you are perfectly aware of it. Take a moment to consider whom you tend to compare yourself to the most often. Is it a friend or relative, or someone on TV or in a magazine? How does this comparison help or hurt you? Keeping your mind on someone else may actually be a way of avoiding your own struggle with food.

On Second Thought: Minding Your Own Plate

Remember that sizing yourself up against someone else is like trying to compare snowflakes. Each snowflake is unique. No two are the same, but all are beautiful. A helpful mind-set is to strive to be the best version of you.

When your mind drifts and starts to envy someone else's body or diet, redirect your thoughts to yourself. Be mindful of your movements. For example, put your palms together and rub them quickly. Notice the heat and friction you create in doing so. Or, place your hands against a table. Draw your attention to the sensation of the space between your hands and the table. Is it smooth, rough, cool? The point is to notice how you and your body interface with the world. Your body, not someone else's, is what's important. These mindful movements can remind you that you only have control over the sensations within *you*.

If you get down on yourself because you are stuck in comparisons, turn your attention to your strengths. Reinforce this by applying self-acceptance. Tell yourself *I am enough, just as I am.* If you have particularly aggressive and competitive backseat-driver thoughts, be more directive with your thoughts. When mindless thoughts seep into your consciousness, kindly and calmly respond *I am minding my own body.*

43. *I'm Not Buying These Cookies for Me* Thoughts

My relationship with food is like a game of Truth or Dare. Sometimes I tell myself the truth. I'm honest about my true motivation. I tell myself Fast food is terrible for me, but it tastes so good, and I want it. At other times, I just can't face the truth. I dare myself Take just one bite. I tell myself I can just take a nibble and walk away. Deep down I know this is just not true.

—Julia

Julia confessed that she "blew" her diet. She told herself *I'll buy ice cream just for my kids. I don't want any.* Then, she ended up eating half her daughter's cone, and breaking down and getting a scoop for herself. She admitted that it simply wasn't true that she didn't want any. Deep down she knew she longed for ice cream. It was hard to be honest with herself about this craving.

Perhaps you know what this is like. Maybe you've said to yourself *I'll buy these cookies to save for a special occasion,* knowing full well you wouldn't be able to stay away from them. You ate a few cookies here and there, and before you knew it, the entire box was gone. Or, you've thought *I buy these snacks for my husband because he likes them and I don't want to punish him with my dieting,* when in truth he would benefit from eating healthier as well. Why aren't you totally honest with yourself? Why do you tell yourself what you want to hear when, deep down, you know the truth?

Sigmund Freud, the founder of psychoanalysis, was one of the first to explore the many ways we defend against things that don't make us happy. We use defense mechanisms like denial to cope with the reality of a situation and to protect our self-image, but this is also a way to distance ourselves from full awareness of unpleasant thoughts or feelings. Concerning food, you may be protecting yourself from self-judgment. Maybe you know you would verbally beat yourself up if you were honest with yourself about wanting an ice cream cone.

Do any of these defense mechanisms sound familiar?

- **Denial:** Being unaware that there's a problem. *I don't eat mindlessly. My weight isn't a problem.*

- **Reaction formation:** Appearing to be okay with a problem when you aren't. *I'm fine with the way I eat.*

- **Projection:** Placing your undesirable thoughts or feelings onto another person who doesn't have those thoughts. A person may say to his wife, "You eat too much junk food," when really he is concerned about his own eating.

- **Compartmentalization:** Separating your awareness of an issue to the point of behaving as if they were separate values. *My eating doesn't have anything to do with my weight. I'm perfectly healthy. My diabetes isn't really related to what I eat.*

- **Displacement:** Taking your frustration or anger out on another person. *I have to help my daughter* *lose weight* (when really you are angry at yourself for having difficulty managing your weight).

- **Compensation:** Counterbalancing areas of weakness with areas of strength. *I may not be good at eating well, but I exercise every day.*

If you find yourself using any defense mechanisms, it's time to take a closer look at why your mind struggles so hard to keep the reality of the situation at bay.

On Second Thought: Mindful Honesty

Honesty helps you make more-mindful decisions. When you know the truth, you can plan how to handle it. It's like lying to your doctor about a problem because you fear judgment. The doctor can't form a treatment plan that will help you until you reveal the real story. Being less judgmental of your cravings may help you to be more honest with yourself.

To learn how to speak in a nonjudgmental tone, try using a strategy suggested by one of my clients. She modeled her tone after her Global Positioning System (GPS), the kind she used in her car. A GPS tells you which direction to go. When you turn the wrong direction or miss an exit, it says in an even tone, "Recalculating." The tone is matter of fact and devoid of judgment. Practice speaking calmly and rationally, without insult or commentary. This might be difficult and may take practice. When you feel as if you've made a "mistake" with food, delete the commentary and, using a calm and even tone, like a GPS, guide yourself back on track. When you catch yourself using the backseat-driver version—*You shouldn't have eaten that! How could you have been so stupid!*—aim instead for the GPS version by practicing telling yourself in an even and toneless manner:

- *Next time, I'll make a better choice.*

- *That wasn't the best choice, but it isn't the end of the world.*

- *I can get back on track.*

- *I can start again.*

If you can, take it one step further. After you've mastered the neutral voice, speak to yourself with compassion. Initiate statements to yourself with kind words:

- *It's hard...*

- *It must be a painful decision...*

- *You are really wrestling with this problem...*

44. *If I Eat Well Now, I Can Have a Cookie Later* Thought

I ate so mindfully this week. I didn't cheat at all. I'm going to reward myself with ice cream.

—Tom

Tom promised himself a scoop of chocolate ice cream if he packed his lunch with healthy foods all week. It sounds like a wise idea to give yourself a prize for taking steps toward mindful eating. But, rewarding yourself with food, or even other gifts, may actually make the problem worse instead of better.

Token gifts or external rewards are a type of extrinsic rewards. *Extrinsic rewards*, like money, grades, and good food, are given to increase your motivation to repeat a particular behavior. *Intrinsic rewards*, by contrast, are the internal rewards that come from doing something well, and they include feeling joyful, successful, competent, or proud. Think of one of your hobbies, like knitting. No one pays you to knit a sweater. You are motivated to do it because you enjoy it. If someone offered to pay you money to do it, suddenly there would be a new dynamic and reason for doing it. It probably would take some of the joy out of it and harm your motivation. The reward isn't in the money; it's in the process and challenge of seeing the sweater come together.

When your mind tries to play *Let's Make a Deal*, be cautious about how you respond. For example, if you tell yourself *If I avoid sugar all day today, I'll buy a cookie tomorrow*, pause for a moment. Remind yourself of the difference between extrinsic and intrinsic motivation. The cookie is extrinsic, a reward outside of yourself. This kind of reward won't increase the likelihood that you will continue to work on reducing your sugar intake. Once the cookie is eaten, its reinforcement value is over. Your motivation will probably fall flat, because once you reach the "carrot," you stop. Remember that you are more likely to continue your efforts to change your eating if you don't give yourself too many external rewards, even though it's very tempting. Feeling healthy *is* the reward. We are so accustomed to giving ourselves gifts that we come to expect tangible rewards and feel that we deserve them.

On Second Thought: Mindfully Feeling Good

Learning to draw your awareness to the benefits or intrinsic rewards that come from eating well will keep your motivation going much longer than an external reward of food, money, or trinkets.

Notice the natural rewards you get from eating well. Say you cut down on eating refined sugar for an entire day. At the end of the day, take a moment to appreciate the natural benefits to your body and mood. Maybe you noticed you had more energy, because your blood sugar remained stable. Perhaps you felt more even keeled and less moody. Closely observing and zooming in on such internal rewards will help you avoid sugar again tomorrow. Mindful eaters eat well because it naturally feels good, not because they get a special gift in return.

Make healthy eating a hobby, or increase the intrinsic value of doing it. Ask yourself *What part of healthy eating do I naturally find enjoyable?* If you are a gardener, planting healthy foods might give you great amounts of joy. If you like to cook, searching for cookbooks with healthy recipes at the bookstore can keep you entertained for hours. Love to shop? Find a good health-food store to browse at your leisure. Again, this increases the intrinsic reward associated with eating well.

45. *I'm So Fat* Thoughts

I worry a lot about my teenaged daughter getting bullied. I don't want anyone calling her names or tearing down her self-esteem. The other day, my daughter was snacking in the kitchen, and I heard her say to her friend, "I shouldn't be eating this; it's so bad! I'm so fat and ugly." I was so worried that other people would bully my daughter that I didn't even realize she was bullying herself.

—Zoe

Fogging (Smith 1975) is a classic assertiveness technique I often teach my clients. You can use this technique to challenge a bully, such as a verbally abusive coworker or an angry spouse. It confuses your opponent so that the person often stops bothering you.

How does fogging work? A bully expects and tries to coax you into fighting back. This type of person likes getting under your skin to feel powerful. Instead of engaging you in battle, fogging strategically uses agreement, which a bully doesn't expect. Instead of disagreeing with a critical statement, agree with the part that's true or possibly true. This harmonizes with the concept of mindfulness, because you aren't struggling against the thought or idea. You don't get into an argument with backseat-driver thoughts.

Fogging can work well in dealing with your inner critic. The inner self-critic tries to poke at you so that you fight back. Perhaps you have gotten into a verbal argument with your inner critic. Your inner critic says you are *bad* or *stupid* for blowing your diet, so you fight back with things like *I'm not stupid*. The debate gets heated and continues back and forth. Fogging is a way of side-stepping the mental battle.

On Second Thought: Fogging It Out

The next time you verbally beat yourself up, try this mindful fogging technique.

1. **Critical thought:** *I can't believe I ate that sweet roll. It's so fattening. I blew it again! How could I be so weak?*

2. **Initial temptation:** *I'm not weak. I didn't completely blow it!* This engages your mind in a fight. Getting sucked into an argument moves you away from taking productive action.

3. **Mindful response using fogging:** *It's true that I ate the sweet roll. It probably isn't the best option, because it isn't the healthiest. I can do better. It wasn't my finest moment. Next time I'll do better.*

Notice how this diffuses the intensity and shame the inner critic wishes to bestow on you.

46. *I Can't Stand It* Thoughts

I hate looking in the mirror. I can't stand it! Every day I feel so uncomfortable and desperate to get this weight off my body. My desperation hasn't done me any favors. You wouldn't believe the things I've tried to lose weight—crazy crash diets. I've spent more money on worthless products than you can imagine and stuffed myself into clothes I couldn't breathe in.

—Erin

Uncomfortable feelings are like airplane turbulence. They jolt you around and cause a lot of discomfort and sometimes even panic. Consider for a moment how you would cope with severe turbulence. Would you reassure yourself that it will stop? Distract yourself by talking to the person next to you? Pray? Ignore it? Maybe you would use facts to rationalize the situation, such as remind yourself that planes are the safest way to travel.

How you talk yourself through things like airplane turbulence and other stressful situations you can't control or don't think you can "stand" is indicative of your coping strategies. It gives you a snapshot of the self-dialogue you naturally use to cope with stressful situations. The good thing about airplane turbulence is that it's an exercise in endurance. There's nothing you can do to escape it except calm yourself until the turbulence is over.

On Second Thought: Finding Endurance

Try this experiment. If you are physically able, stand on one foot. You can probably do this with ease for a few seconds. As time slips by, you are bound to get a bit fatigued. Perhaps your foot muscles begin to get heavy. Notice what's happening in your mind. It probably resorts to backseat-driver thoughts like *I can't take this; I really want to put my foot down.* Eventually, *I can't stand this* may pop into your mind. Tell yourself *Just another minute.* This opens up an opportunity to build your endurance. When your mind wants to convince you that changing your eating is too difficult to bear, respond mindfully.

Backseat-Driver Thoughts	**Mindful Response**
I can't do this; it's too hard.	*Just stick with it another moment.*
I can't stand it.	*I don't like it, but I can endure it and cope without my thoughts making it worse.*
When will this stop?	*It's not a big deal; I can take it a little longer.*
This is awful.	*It doesn't feel good, but I can handle this.*
Ugh, it's unbearable.	*It won't kill me. I can do it.*

47. *It's My Family's Fault That I'm Overweight* Thoughts

I blame the way I eat on my mother. She's such a food pusher. Even as an adult, she says, "Have another bite," even after I've clearly said, "No thank you." She'll tell you, "That's what Italian grandmothers do."

—Vicky

Vicky wasn't invited to her friend Sara's birthday party. For weeks, she waited for an invitation, and as each week passed, she began coming up with possible reasons why she wasn't invited and dwelling on each: *I must have said something to offend her* or *We must not really be friends.* Each day she got angrier and more sullen. In the parking lot, she ignored Sara's waves. Vicky began calling herself a "loser" for not getting invited. The day before Sara's party, Vicky picked up a pile of old mail, and an invitation that had been stuck between two magazines fell to the floor.

Like Vicky, we all create stories about our experiences and who we are. It's easy to get caught up in believing these stories without question. The story affects how you feel and, in turn, how you act.

We do a lot of storytelling about our hunger and weight. We create stories about the way we eat, particularly about who or what is to "blame" for our eating habits. And, we hold firmly to why it's difficult or impossible to eat healthier, cope with cravings, and lose weight: *No one in my family is at a healthy weight, I have a slow metabolism,* or *I can't manage my weight because I'm addicted to sugar.* Perhaps your story includes self-blame or blame of others: *My mother was a food pusher* or *My husband is always buying unhealthy food.*

It's true that many of these factors can make change extremely difficult. Your spouse probably isn't making it any easier to eat healthy. And you might have an extreme sensitivity to sugar. But sometimes it's simply the story that keeps you stuck. When you try to do something new, the backseat driver pops up and directs you back to acting in accordance with the story's script.

A mindful approach doesn't seek blame. It gravitates toward understanding and seeing these thoughts for what they are—just a story. The script doesn't determine what you can or cannot do.

On Second Thought: Mentally Step Back

Consider whether you tell any stories about how you eat. How do these stories keep you trapped? Who or what do you blame when you overeat?

Try mentally taking a step back from the center of the story. In other words, instead of telling your story from within the story, use a different vantage point. Imagine that you are a friend or a movie narrator, or that you are watching yourself on a movie screen. When you watch your "movie," observe what's happening from a distance. What part of your story keeps you stuck?

48. *I'll Be Happy When I Lose Weight* Thoughts

I get stuck in this dilemma: I'll feel better about myself when I lose weight, but I can't lose weight until I feel better about myself. *So then I do absolutely nothing.*

—Jeff

What would you do if you won the lottery? Buy a house, retire, go on vacation? We all think *I'd finally be happy if I won the lottery.*

Jeff won a great sum of money. To everyone's surprise, one year after collecting his new fortune, he was severely depressed. Money couldn't fix his fractured relationship with his kids or help him lose weight. Stories about lottery winners reveal an interesting picture. Sometimes people tend to return to the same level of happiness as before they won the money, just like Jeff. If you were a very unhappy person prior to winning the lottery, you are probably just as unhappy afterward.

If you lost all the weight you wanted to, you'd probably feel as if you had won the lottery. Losing weight will definitely contribute to your health and happiness, but it won't make everything magically better, as we often believe it will. The bottom line is that your thoughts put too much pressure on you when you hold this belief, making happiness a "make it or break it" situation that requires you to lose weight to feel good.

On Second Thought: Happiness Now

Notice when you hear your mind say *I'll be happy when…* (in this case, *when I've lost weight*). Give yourself a little mental nudge. Rather than thinking of a global sense of happiness, refocus your mind to specific things you'll gain, like a healthier weight, fitting better into your clothes, having a lower cholesterol level. Instead of *I'll be happy when I lose weight*, tell yourself *What makes me happy about this journey today* (or *in this moment*) *is…* (*fitting into my smaller clothes this morning, how good I felt after I ate a healthy snack*, and so on).

From a mindful perspective, all you have is the "now." You've already arrived at this very moment. Now is the good part of life. List silently or out loud three things that make you happy right now in your journey toward more-mindful eating. Your new mantra is *I have everything I need to be happy now*. Repeat it to yourself whenever you feel a little blue about your weight or eating habits.

49. *I Can't Stop Thinking about Food* Thoughts

I'm so bad. I think about food morning, noon, and night. While I'm supposed to be working or listening to my wife, in the very back of my mind, I'm contemplating what to eat next. I don't know why I can't stop thinking about food.

—Chris

Sometimes I give my clients homework. One such assignment is to notice how much time they spend thinking about food. To help them get to the bottom of this, I often send my clients home with a worksheet containing an empty circle that they will turn into a pie chart. I ask them to just observe the content of their thoughts for one day, noticing what they think about, such as their jobs, kids, bills, eating, and so on. Then, the next step is to draw a pie chart representing roughly how much time they spend thinking about each category. This exercise is often pretty telling about a person's relationship with food.

We all have to spend a reasonable amount of time thinking about food: planning snacks and where to get the next meal. But, when someone reports thinking about food for more than half the day, this is a red flag indicating a deeper issue. The person often ruminates or obsesses about food, like a hamster going around and around a wheel. Some clients say, "Food is always in the back of my mind," "I always find myself scheming about good things I can find to eat," or "I find my mind drifting off, and suddenly I'm daydreaming about something yummy."

When people with very problematic eating habits complete the worksheet, the majority of the circle is filled with thoughts about food. They say things like, "I am obsessively thinking about food." It's this annoying thing that constantly tugs on them.

On Second Thought: Get Out of Your Head

Notice when you are dwelling on food thoughts. Tell yourself *I'm obsessing about food again.* Catch yourself red handed. You may notice that your eyes are fuzzy or that you have moved into a daydream-like state.

Walk mindfully. When you obsess about food, you focus only on things happening from the neck up. To disengage from your thoughts, reinhabit your body. Take a walk down the hallway. Draw all your attention to your feet. Notice how they touch the floor. Hear the rhythm of your walking. Redirect your focus onto your body. Maybe you have experienced this during physical intimacy. When you think too much, you don't feel the sensations.

Hum. If you just can't disengage your mind from food cravings, find something else to ruminate about, like a catchy phrase from a commercial or some song lyrics. You know the kind that you just can't get out of your head. While that's often annoying, you can use it to your advantage in certain circumstances.

Engage in well-timed thinking. Allow yourself a specific amount of time to think about food and your eating habits. Tell yourself *I'll think about this again later.* Dedicating time to nothing else but thinking about food will help you to stop obsessing about food when you need to be focused on something else. Be sure to choose a time when you aren't too hungry, to avoid increasing your ruminating.

Check your hunger. Thinking about food a lot may be caused by excessive hunger. When you restrict your food too much or don't eat enough healthy, filling whole foods, your mind thinks about food to signal you that you need to eat. Consider whether you are eating enough whole, nourishing foods.

50. *I Don't Want Eating to Be a Problem* Thoughts

I don't want eating to be a problem. Eating should be easy, fun, and enjoyable. The last time I really felt like that was when I was a kid. I don't want to think or worry about it anymore. I flip-flop between This is a problem for me *and* I don't want this to be a problem. *Stewing about this keeps me stuck. I put off dealing with it for another day.*

—Andrea

Several years ago, Andrea told me a story about getting lost. She got on a train in a small town in northern Italy and headed for Venice. Somewhere along the way, she nodded off, and eventually, the conductor began shaking her. The train had stopped at a station, and Andrea got off. For several minutes, she was disoriented. This was not Venice. For ten minutes, she stewed about the situation. The train ticket said "Venice." *This* has *to be it* she told herself. She didn't want to be somewhere else. Exiting the train anywhere besides her intended destination would make things infinitely more difficult. Once she realized she had missed her stop, there was a part of her that just couldn't face it. To come up with a plan, she had to accept where she was rather than insist that she was where she wanted to be.

Starting from where you are with your eating may be difficult for this very reason. It's not where you want to be or think you "should" be. Maybe you think *I should be wearing a smaller size right now* or *I should be further along with changing my eating.* You can't make a plan until you truly accept, in an open and nonjudgmental way, where you are right now.

Accepting your thoughts is challenging. Sometimes you don't like what they have to say. You may have a thought and then twist it all around, trying to make it into something new or different. Wrestling with your mind takes you out of the present. The following are some ways you may show nonacceptance of your thoughts:

- Judging thoughts. *How could I think something so dumb?*

- Arguing or debating thoughts. *No, that isn't true. I don't deserve to be healthier.*

- Questioning or pondering whether thoughts are true. *Could it be true? Is my mother right that I need to lose weight?*

- Overanalyzing or picking apart thoughts, such as thinking about a thought too long when it doesn't mean anything. *I wonder if I really shouldn't eat that? Does it really matter? Will one or two bites really make that much difference?*

- Wishing the thoughts away. *I wish I didn't think about food so much! If only I could just stop thinking about what I'm going to eat all the time!*

- Agreeing with or validating the thoughts. *That's true; I'm terrible at watching my weight.*

- Ignoring the thoughts or pretending you didn't think them. *That doughnut isn't good for me! I can't think about that right now.*

- Pushing the thoughts away or telling yourself not to think that way. *Stop it! Stop thinking such negative things about yourself.*

- Confirming the truth, or looking around yourself in search of evidence to back up your thoughts. *See, it must be true, because…*

These strategies often leave you wrestling with your thoughts. Don't try to maneuver your thoughts into something else or change them.

On Second Thought: It Is What It Is

When you notice your mind playing tug-of-war with your thoughts, imagine stepping away from the struggle. Label what you are doing: "analyzing," "denying," "fighting," and so on. Then, let go by telling yourself *It is what it is. Accept; don't change.* Allow yourself to accept that food issues are difficult.

Chapter 5

A Day in the Life
of a Mindful Eater

One question you may have is how to put together all the information in this book. Let's meet Betsy and follow her for one day. She's a good example of how often counterproductive thoughts pop up in a twenty-four-hour period. Betsy is a teacher who lives with her ailing mother. She has a very stressful life. Let's examine how Betsy uses mindfulness techniques to deal with self-sabotaging thoughts.

6:30 a.m. Waking Up

Betsy is lying in bed. As her eyes open, her mind begins to race. Her very first thoughts are about food. She says to herself *Oh great, your feet haven't even hit the floor and you're already thinking about food!* but then catches herself: *Betsy, that's a judgment*, and softly reminds herself that she needs to simply observe the thought (see chapter 4, thought 31). When Betsy is tempted to judge herself, she allows the thought to come and go. She uses her GPS voice to respond calmly and graciously (see chapter 4, thought 43). She decides to take things one moment at a time.

7:00 a.m. Getting Ready

Betsy scans her bedroom closet, and a feeling of dread arises. What would she wear? Hopeless thoughts like *I can't stand this* and *Why bother?* begin flooding her mind. Betsy recalls the tips she learned in this book and reminds herself of how to deal with thoughts of desperation and hopelessness. Betsy reassures herself: *I can do this. It will take time* (see chapter 4, thought 46).

8:00 a.m. Breakfast

Betsy's mother sits at the kitchen table eating muffins covered with brown sugar and butter. Betsy acknowledges her feeling of temptation and desire. *I have no willpower* is the first thought that enters her mind. Betsy gives herself a little mental nudge and reminds herself: *Willpower is not a magical skill. It's something that develops with time and practice* (see chapter 4, thought 34). She decides to use this situation as a skill-building exercise: *Instead of the muffin, I choose something else that I know will be healthier, more filling, and empowering to my body.* She picks Greek yogurt, because it has a lot of protein. *Food is medicine*, she reminds herself (see chapter 3, thought 22).

9:00 a.m. Teachers' Conference

As soon as she arrives at the teachers' conference, Betsy is greeted with a delicious-looking spread of goodies. Mindlessly, she picks up a doughnut and starts nervously munching on it. Suddenly, she realizes what she is doing. Her detour thoughts say *You already started the doughnut; why not finish? It's too late; you ruined it anyway.*

Betsy typically falls hook, line, and sinker for this kind of excuse. But now, she returns her focus to the moment by watching that thought come and letting it exit her mind as if it were walking out the door (see chapter 3, thought 2). *I'm having an all-or-nothing thought*, she realizes, immediately throwing away the rest of the doughnut so that she isn't tempted to graze on it. Then, she gets a cup of coffee to keep her hands busy (see chapter 3, thought 9).

10:00 a.m. Midmorning

Before the meeting ends, a teacher passes around a plate of homemade cookies. Two thoughts run through Betsy's mind: *I must have one!* and *If I eat that, I'll ruin my diet.* She responds *The day isn't ruined just because I ate something mindlessly. Each action is a choice* (see chapter 3, thought 2). Betsy reminds herself that she has many more choices to make during the day. She looks at each of these decisions as an opportunity to do better. *No, thank you,* she says to herself. She practiced saying a "powerful no" so that she'd be ready when tempted by treats (see chapter 4, thought 33). The teacher who made the cookies continues to urge her to take one. Betsy politely smiles, takes one, wraps it in a napkin and says, "Thank you. I'll eat it later." As soon as she returns to her classroom, she immediately gives the cookie to a friend so she won't nibble on it later.

12:00 Noon Lunchtime

Betsy balances her tray on her forearm as she walks through the cafeteria line. *I shouldn't eat that* keeps playing through her mind as she looks at different lunch options. Instead of creating a "should" rule, she asks herself *Is that sandwich really what my body wants?* As this book advises (see chapter 4, thought 35), she responds to "should" by rephrasing the statement to view her decisions in the context of mindful eating.

1:00 p.m. Afternoon

Betsy starts ruminating about food even though she just finished lunch. *Am I really hungry?* she asks herself (see chapter 3, thought 6). The leftover food in the conference room seems to call her name. She welcomes this message and asks herself *Do I need a snack?* (See chapter 3, thought 15.) Instead of focusing on what she "can't" have, she instead views the situation from a different perspective, thinking *What would be healthy?* (See chapter 3, thought 3.) Betsy chooses a mindful snack. She keeps apples and granola bars handy in her classroom to prevent her from using the vending machine and buying things on impulse.

4:00 p.m. Late Afternoon

School is over. Betsy's day has been more stressful than usual. The students were uncooperative, and an unhappy parent cornered her. *I need chocolate to comfort myself. I deserve it*, her mind keeps repeating. Betsy often has difficulty managing such thoughts. It has been so easy and habitual to turn to food for comfort. She turns to other calming activities (see chapter 3, thought 27). Immediately, she runs through a prepared list of other soothing options that she has written down: *I could choose a cup of hot tea.* Betsy reassures herself that if the tea doesn't work, she can always go back to the chocolate. Restricting and forbidding herself leads to cravings. To quiet her mind and reduce her stress level naturally and without food, she gives herself permission to take a five-minute mental break, which includes leaning back in her chair, closing her eyes, and taking a few deep, slow breaths (see chapter 3, thought 28).

6:00 p.m. Early Evening

After dinner, Betsy thinks it's the perfect time to go for a walk, but detour thoughts start seducing her with other plans: *Go tomorrow. You don't feel like it now. You're too tired. You've had a rough day.*

Betsy remembers that she just needs to get the ball rolling to combat inertia. To buy into the idea of exercising, she asks herself to start with just a small request: *Just get your shoes on and see how you feel* (see chapter 3, thought 10). Betsy's mind easily agrees that she can grant herself this tiny request. Once her shoes are on, she says to herself *That wasn't so bad; could I just walk to my car? If I feel like doing more, great; if not, that's okay.* Once she passes her car, she makes a slightly larger request of herself: *Just twenty more feet, and I'll be on the walking trail.* Betsy successfully overcomes the urge to procrastinate by taking small steps right now.

7:30 p.m. Evening

Betsy sits down with her mother to watch TV, which is their nightly ritual. They usually bring out the chocolate-brownie ice cream, with each digging into her own pint. Betsy starts craving ice cream and is tempted to get it while she tells her mother about her day. Betsy continues to think about the ice cream, so she takes a proactive step. She gets out her knitting and uses distraction to get her mind off snacking (see chapter 3, thought 27).

9:30 p.m. Nighttime

It's time to take a shower, and the temptation to get on the scale is overwhelming. When Betsy is honest with herself, she realizes this is only her mind trying to set up expectations. The backseat-driver thoughts say *You should've lost two pounds by now.* Getting on the scale is an emotional trap, because the numbers always ignite a flurry of chatter in her head. Betsy berates herself if the number on the scale is higher than she expects. At other times, she is tempted to reward herself with food if the numbers are down. Her mind says *You deserve a treat; you did well.*

Betsy shifts her focus from looking at the numbers to being mindful of her diet and exercise (see chapter 3, thought 17). She knows that if she eats mindfully, the weight will come off in its own time. She goes to bed early. Getting adequate sleep is her greatest ally in skillfully responding to her detour and backseat-driver thoughts (see chapter 3, thought 25). Before she closes her eyes, she thinks *Tomorrow, I will continue to work on eating mindfully and responding consciously to my thoughts.*

References

Barnes, R. D., and S. Tantleff-Dunn. 2010. "Food for Thought: Examining the Relationship between Food Thought Suppression and Weight-Related Outcomes." *Eating Behaviors* 11 (3):175–79.

Basu, A., M. Rhone, and T. J. Lyons. 2010. "Berries: Emerging Impact on Cardiovascular Health." *Nutrition Reviews* 68 (3):168–77.

Defilippis, A. P., M. J. Blaha, and T. A. Jacobson. 2010. "Omega-3 Fatty Acids for Cardiovascular Disease Prevention." *Current Treatment Options in Cardiovascular Medicine* 12 (4):365–80.

Flood-Obbagy, J. E., and B. J. Rolls. 2009. "The Effect of Fruit in Different Forms on Energy Intake and Satiety at a Meal." *Appetite* 52 (2):416–22.

Freedman, D. H. 2011. "How to Fix the Obesity Crisis." *Scientific American* 304 (2):40–47.

Freedman, J. L., and S. C. Fraser. 1966. "Compliance without Pressure: The Foot-in-the-Door Technique." *Journal of Personality and Social Psychology* 4(2):195–202.

Hayes, S. C., K. D. Strosahl, and K. G. Wilson. 1999. *Acceptance and Commitment Therapy: An Experiential Approach to Behavior Change.* New York: The Guilford Press.

Kabat-Zinn, J. 1990. *Full Catastrophe Living: Using the Wisdom of Your Body and Mind to Face Stress, Pain, and Illness.* New York: Delacorte Press.

Linehan, M. M. 1993. *Cognitive-Behavioral Treatment of Borderline Personality Disorder.* New York: The Guilford Press.

Mischel, W., and B. Underwood. 1974. "Instrumental Ideation in Delay of Gratification." *Child Development* 45 (4):1083–88.

Poslusna, K., J. Ruprich, J. H. de Vries, M. Jakubikova, and P. van't Veer. 2009. "Misreporting of Energy and Micronutrient Intake Estimated by Food Records and 24 Hour Recalls, Control and Adjustment Methods in Practice." *British Journal of Nutrition* 101 (Suppl. 2):S73–S85.

Six, B. L., T. E. Schap, F. M. Zhu, A. Mariappan, M. Bosch, E. J. Delp, D. S. Ebert, D. A. Kerr, and C. J. Boushey. 2010. "Evidence-Based Development of a Mobile Telephone Food Record." *Journal of the American Dietetic Association* 110 (1):74–79.

Smith, M. J. 1975. *When I Say No, I Feel Guilty.* New York: Bantam Books.

Tapper, K., C. Shaw, J. Ilsley, A. J. Hill, F. W. Bond, and L. Moore. 2009. "Exploratory Randomised Controlled Trial of a Mindfulness-Based Weight Loss Intervention for Women." *Appetite* 52 (2):396–404.

Titchener, E. B. 1916. *A Text-Book of Psychology.* New York: The MacMillan Company.

Wansink, B. 2004. "Environmental Factors That Increase the Food Intake and Consumption Volume of Unknowing Consumers." *Annual Review of Nutrition* 24:455–79.

Wansink, B., and P. Chandon. 2006. "Meal Size, Not Body Size, Explains Errors in Estimating the Calorie Content of Meals." *Annals of Internal Medicine* 145 (5) 326–32.

Wansink, B., and J. Sobal. 2007. "Mindless Eating: The 200 Daily Food Decisions We Overlook." *Environment and Behavior* 39 (1):106–23.

Williams, M., J. Teasdale, Z. Segal, and J. Kabat-Zinn. 2007. *The Mindful Way through Depression: Freeing Yourself from Chronic Unhappiness.* New York: The Guilford Press.

Wood, A. M., J. J. Froh, and A. W. A. Geraghty. 2010. "Gratitude and Well-Being: A Review and Theoretical Integration." *Clinical Psychology Review* 30 (7):890–905.

Susan Albers, Psy.D., is a psychologist at the Cleveland Clinic Family Health Center who specializes in eating issues, weight loss, body image concerns and mindfulness. After obtaining a masters and doctorate degree from the University of Denver, Dr. Albers completed an APA internship at the University of Notre Dame in South Bend, Indiana and a post-doctoral fellowship at Stanford University in California. Dr. Albers conducts mindful eating workshops across the country and internationally.

Dr. Albers is the author of *50 Ways to Soothe Yourself Without Food*, *Eating Mindfully*, *Eat, Drink, and Be Mindful* and *Mindful Eating 101*. Her work has been featured in *O, the Oprah Magazine*, *Family Circle*, *Shape*, *Prevention Magazine*, *Self*, *Health*, *Fitness Magazine*, *Vanity Fair*, *Natural Health*, and the *Wall Street Journal*. Susan write a blog for the *Huffington Post* and *Psychology Today*. She has been on many TV shows including being a guest expert on the Dr. Oz, T.V. show.

Dr. Albers is a member of the Academy for Eating Disorders, International Association of Eating Disorder Professionals and the National Eating Disorders Association. Susan enjoys spending time blogging, jogging in 5K races, watching the Sundance Channel, and traveling. Visit Albers online at www.eatingmindfully.com

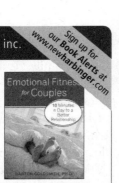
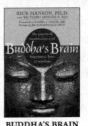
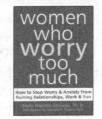
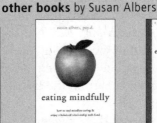
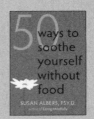
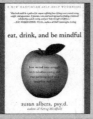